Child and Adolescent Psychiatry

T0323314

What Do I Do Now?—Psychiatry

SERIES EDITOR
Marc Agronin

PUBLISHED AND FORTHCOMING TITLES:

Child and Adolescent Psychiatry by Robyn P. Thom and Christopher J. McDougle

Geriatric Psychiatry By Marc Agronin And Ipsit Vahia

Child and Adolescent Psychiatry

Edited by

Robyn P. Thom, MD
Massachusetts General Hospital
Lurie Center for Autism
Instructor of Psychiatry
Harvard Medical School
Boston, MA, USA

Christopher J. McDougle, MD
Director, Lurie Center for Autism
Massachusetts General Hospital
Department of Psychiatry
Harvard Medical School
Boston, MA, USA

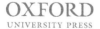

OXFORD
UNIVERSITY PRESS

OXFORD
UNIVERSITY PRESS

Oxford University Press is a department of the University of Oxford. It furthers
the University's objective of excellence in research, scholarship, and education
by publishing worldwide. Oxford is a registered trade mark of Oxford University
Press in the UK and certain other countries.

Published in the United States of America by Oxford University Press
198 Madison Avenue, New York, NY 10016, United States of America.

© Oxford University Press 2021

Library of Congress Cataloging-in-Publication Data
Names: Thom, Robyn P., editor. | McDougle, Christopher J., editor.
Title: Child and adolescent psychiatry / edited by Robyn P. Thom,
Christopher J. McDougle.
Other titles: Child and adolescent psychiatry (Thom) | What do I do now?
Description: New York, NY : Oxford University Press, [2021] |
Series: What do i do now? | Includes bibliographical references and index.
Identifiers: LCCN 2021008100 (print) | LCCN 2021008101 (ebook) |
ISBN 9780197577479 (paperback) | ISBN 9780197577486 (epub) |
ISBN 9780197577509 (online)
Subjects: MESH: Autism Spectrum Disorder | Child | Adolescent |
Case Reports
Classification: LCC RC553.A88 (print) | LCC RC553.A88 (ebook) |
NLM WS 350.8.P4 | DDC 616.85/88200835—dc23
LC record available at https://lccn.loc.gov/2021008100
LC ebook record available at https://lccn.loc.gov/2021008101

DOI: 10.1093/med/9780197577479.001.0001

9 8 7 6 5 4 3 2 1
Printed by Marquis, Canada

Contents

* Faculty advisor

Foreword

Many of us find it helpful when a speaker includes a clinical case to illustrate key teaching points during a lecture. We tend to reorient and recall diagnostic and treatment decisions we made when caring for similar patients. Confirming that our practice approaches are consistent with the standard of care is reassuring. Alternatively, we may acquire new clinical knowledge for a future patient. The *What Do I Do Now?* series of books published by Oxford University Press utilizes this cased-based approach to learning, with volumes addressing various specialty and subspecialty areas in the field of medicine.

The intended readership for the *What Do I Do Now?—Child and Adolescent Psychiatry* book includes medical students, general psychiatry residents, and child and adolescent psychiatry fellows. Who better to write the clinical vignettes and background material than representatives of the targeted audience? Each chapter has been authored by a medical student, general psychiatry resident, or child and adolescent psychiatry fellow in the Harvard Medical School system. The medical students felt that a succinct, clinically relevant chapter would inspire confidence and help develop their psychiatric assessment and treatment planning skills. The general psychiatry residents wanted the content to be useful during a rotation on child and adolescent psychiatry and wanted to learn how their approach to adult psychiatry could be adapted to youth. Each clinical vignette needed to be supported by up-to-date information on epidemiology, signs, and symptoms that define the disorder based on the *Diagnostic and Statistical Manual of Mental Disorders,* Fifth Edition (DSM-5), assessment and recommended biological (including medication management), psychological (including developmental assessment and psychotherapeutic approaches), and social (including cultural, environmental, and educational considerations as well as recommendations and resources for parents [e.g., educational advocacy, self-help groups, and toolkits/facts for families]) treatments. The child and adolescent psychiatry fellows emphasized the importance of taking a developmental perspective and determined that including "Key Points to Remember" and references for further reading should be provided at the end of each chapter.

Certainly, interns in psychology and residents and fellows in neurology, pediatrics, or family medicine with an interest in psychiatric disorders affecting youth will also find the book easy to use, clinically oriented, and evidence based. It is intended to be read and understood during a four- to 12-week rotation focused on child and adolescent psychiatry and during review and preparation for board examinations required throughout professional school and postgraduate training. Parents may also find *What Do I Do Now?—Child and Adolescent Psychiatry* accessible, readable, and pertinent to their child. They may also benefit from the resources meant for parents included in each chapter. If the book sparks your interest in considering a career helping children and adolescents with psychiatric disorders and their families, or advocating for them, even more will have been realized.

Robyn P. Thom, MD
Christopher J. McDougle, MD
Boston, Massachusetts
October 15, 2020

Contributors

Emily Anderberg, PhD
Neuropsychology Fellow
Department of Psychiatry
Massachusetts General Hospital
Woburn, MA, USA

David L. Beckmann, MD, MPH
Staff Psychiatrist
Addiction Recovery Management
   Service
Department of Psychiatry
Massachusetts General Hospital
Boston, MA, USA

Kathryn S. Czepiel, MD
Resident
Department of Pediatrics
Massachusetts General Hospital
N. Attleboro, MA, USA

Lauren N. Deaver, MD
Department of Psychiatry
Massachusetts General Hospital
Somerville, MA, USA

Craig L. Donnelly, MD
Professor of Psychiatry
Department of Psychiatry
Dartmouth-Hitchcock
   Medical Center
Lebanon, NH, USA

Eun Kyung Ellen Kim, MD
Resident
Department of Psychiatry
Massachusetts General Hospital/
   McLean Hospital
Cambridge, MA, USA

Katherine A. Epstein, MD, MA
Resident
Department of Psychiatry
Beth Israel Deaconess
   Medical Center
Boston, MA, USA

Mila N. Grossman, MD
Resident
Department of Psychiatry
Massachusetts General Hospital
Cambridge, MA, USA

Kevin M. Hill, MD
Resident
Department of Psychiatry
Beth Israel Deaconess
   Medical Center
Boston, MA, USA

Alex S. Keuroghlian, MD, MPH
Department of Psychiatry
Massachusetts General Hospital
Associate Professor of Psychiatry
Harvard Medical School
Boston, MA, USA

Christina L. Macenski, MD
Resident
Department of Psychiatry
Brigham and Women's Hospital
Harvard Medical School
Brookline, MA, USA

Christopher J. McDougle, MD
Director, Lurie Center for Autism
Massachusetts General Hospital
Department of Psychiatry
Harvard Medical School
Boston, MA, USA

Sirin Ozdemir, MD
Child Psychiatry Fellow
Massachusetts General Hospital
Department of Psychiatry
Harvard Medical School
Belmont, MA, USA

Joseph A. Pereira, MD
Resident
Department of Psychiatry
Columbia University
Clark, NJ, USA

Cordelia Y. Ross, MD, MS
Child Psychiatry Fellow
Department of Psychiatry
Massachusetts General Hospital
Somerville, MA, USA

Sumita Sharma, MD
Resident
Department of Psychiatry
Beth Israel Deaconess
   Medical Center
Milpitas, CA, USA

Danielle Sipsock, MD
Child & Adolescent Psychiatrist
Center for Autism &
   Developmental Disorders
Maine Behavioral Healthcare
Scarborough, ME, USA

Joshua R. Smith, MD
Child Psychiatry Fellow
Department of Psychiatry
Massachusetts General Hospital
Boston, MA, USA

Samantha M. Taylor, MD
Physician
Department of Psychiatry
Brigham and Women's Hospital
Boston, MA, USA

Robyn P. Thom, MD
Massachusetts General Hospital
Lurie Center for Autism
Instructor of Psychiatry
Harvard Medical School
Boston, MA, USA

Ivana Viani, MD
Department of Psychiatry
Brigham and Women's Hospital
Boston, MA, USA

1 Young boy with social impairment and repetitive behaviors

Sirin Ozdemir and Craig L. Donnelly

A five-year-old boy presents due to challenging behaviors at home and school. At times he becomes physically aggressive, especially when transitioning from one activity to another. Per his teacher, he is mostly indifferent to peers, initiates conversations infrequently, but mostly seems to be "stuck in his own world." He is a picky eater, cannot have tags in his clothes, and is hypersensitive to loud noises. He has a very intense interest in the presidents of the United States and often repeats their names to himself in chronological order. On psychiatric assessment, he answers questions with a few words but does not spontaneously share information or initiate conversation. He cannot sustain eye contact. When the psychiatrist offers him a toy car, he becomes excited, makes a screeching sound, and starts flapping his hands. He then starts turning the wheels of the car instead of engaging in pretend play and seems to be fascinated with the spinning motion.

What Do You Do Now?

The patient's presentation is consistent with autism spectrum disorder (ASD), a neurodevelopmental disorder characterized by persistent deficits in social communication and social interaction as well as restricted, repetitive patterns of behavior, interests, or activities. Children with ASD require a variety of behavioral, medical, educational, and other therapeutic services. Therefore, the timely identification of ASD and diagnosis of co-occurring mental and physical disorders is critical for providing evidence-based interventions early in development. Introducing these interventions during the first few years of life can reduce the severity of the core and associated symptoms of ASD, help children achieve developmental milestones, and improve the overall quality of life for children with ASD and their families.

EPIDEMIOLOGY

According to the Centers for Disease Control and Prevention (CDC), approximately 1 in 59 children in the United States is estimated to have ASD. Autism spectrum disorder is approximately four times more common in males than in females. The likelihood of a diagnosis of ASD in the sibling of a child with idiopathic ASD (no known causative medical condition or genetic syndrome) is approximately 10% to 20%.

More than 70% of individuals with ASD have a concurrent medical, developmental, or other psychiatric disorder. Approximately 45% of children with ASD have accompanying intellectual disability (ID), 50% have attention-deficit/hyperactivity disorder (ADHD), and 30% have a seizure disorder. A specific genetic cause of ASD can be identified in about 15% of individuals, most commonly in patients with global developmental delay, ID, and/or dysmorphic features.

Autism spectrum disorder is a complex disorder resulting from the combination of genetic and environmental factors, affecting children of all racial, ethnic, and socioeconomic groups. Factors that increase a child's risk for ASD include advanced parental age, a sibling with ASD, history of prematurity, fetal exposure to valproate, maternal infection during pregnancy, and closer spacing of pregnancies. Some of the known genetic causes of ASD include Fragile X syndrome, tuberous sclerosis complex, 15q11-13 maternal duplications, and 16p11.2 duplications or deletions. Immunizations have not been found to increase the risk of ASD.

SIGNS AND SYMPTOMS

According to the *Diagnostic and Statistical Manual of Mental Disorders*, Fifth Edition (DSM-5), ASD is characterized by persistent deficits in two symptom domains: social communication and interaction as well as restricted, repetitive patterns of behavior, interests, or activities. To qualify for a diagnosis of ASD, individuals must exhibit either current or past social deficits in the three areas of social-emotional reciprocity (e.g., abnormal social approach, failure of back-and-forth conversation, reduced sharing of interests or emotions, failure to respond to or initiate social interactions); nonverbal communicative behaviors used for social interaction (e.g., poorly integrated verbal and nonverbal communication, abnormalities in eye contact and body language, deficits in understanding gestures, lack of nonverbal communication); and developing, maintaining, and understanding relationships (e.g., difficulty adjusting behavior to suit various social contexts, difficulty sharing in imaginative play, decreased or no interest in peers). The individual must also exhibit at least two restricted, repetitive patterns of behavior, interests, or activities manifesting as stereotyped or repetitive motor movements, use of objects, or speech; insistence on sameness/resistance to change; highly restricted, fixated interests that are abnormal in intensity or focus; and hyper- or hyporeactivity to sensory input or unusual interest in sensory aspects of the environment. These symptoms must be present in early development; however, there is no age threshold for making the diagnosis, since symptoms may not be clinically significant until social demands exceed the individual's abilities.

Based on the DSM-5 classification of ASD, there are three levels of severity, which should be assessed separately for social communication and restricted, repetitive behaviors (Level 1: Requiring support, Level 2: Requiring substantial support, and Level 3: Requiring very substantial support). The DSM-5 also includes specifiers for the presence or absence of associated conditions including intellectual impairment, language impairment, catatonia, and known medical, genetic, or environmental factors.

ASSESSMENT

Individuals with ASD may present for clinical assessment at any point in development for a variety of developmental and behavioral problems associated with ASD. There are no laboratory tests or biomarkers to diagnose ASD. A thorough assessment of the child's developmental history, behavioral history obtained from the patient and caregivers, reports of behavior in other environments (such as school), and descriptions of behavior during formal testing is the gold standard for diagnosis. Obtaining the history of symptoms of ASD can be supported by using questionnaires such as the Social Communication Questionnaire (SCQ) or the Social Responsiveness Scale (SRS) and validated observation tools like the Autism Diagnostic Observation Schedule, Second Edition (ADOS-2). While neuropsychological tests and rating scales are not sufficient to make the diagnosis of ASD, they may provide a structured approach to inform the diagnostic application of the DSM-5 criteria.

A comprehensive evaluation for ASD ideally should be completed by a multidisciplinary team including a specialist who has expertise in the diagnosis and management of ASD such as a developmental-behavioral pediatrician, child psychiatrist, or child neurologist. Other providers, however, such as general pediatricians or child psychologists who are familiar with the presentation of ASD and the DSM-5 criteria can also make an initial clinical diagnosis. Other members of the multidisciplinary team may include a neuropsychologist, geneticist and/or genetic counselor, physical therapist, occupational therapist, and speech and language therapist. Formal assessments of the child's language ability, adaptive functioning, neurocognitive profile, and sensory profile are also important components of the diagnostic process.

Features of the mental status examination of a child with ASD may include poor eye contact, difficulty with joint attention and turn taking, deficits in responding to people's emotions/facial expressions or gestures, and limited amount of spontaneously shared experiences. The child may engage in repetitive, ritualistic behaviors or stereotypies. A stereotypy is a purposeless, non-goal-directed, rhythmic, continuous movement, typically manifesting in the upper extremities bilaterally. It can be used to relieve emotions that differ from the baseline mood state such as irritability, anxiety, anger, or excitement. They are voluntary movements that occur in clusters, appear multiple times per day, and last for seconds to minutes. Examples of stereotypies commonly seen in ASD include hand flapping, arm flapping, finger wiggling, running objects across one's peripheral vision, body rocking, and toe walking. Children with ASD may also demonstrate peculiar linguistic tendencies, including a pedantic style, awkward tone and rate (e.g., robotic speech), and echolalia (meaningless repetition of another person's speech), and may show deficits in maintaining a reciprocal conversation. Incorrect use of pronouns, for example, saying, "You want to go outside" or "He wants to go outside" instead of "I want to go outside," is also common. Body language, facial expressions, and nonverbal communication may be awkward and inappropriate.

The diagnostic interview should include a detailed review of the developmental history, assessment for the presence of common medical conditions associated with ASD (e.g., gastrointestinal problems, seizures, sleep disorder, ear infections) and common psychiatric conditions associated with ASD (e.g., tics, ADHD, anxiety), family history (including history of ID, genetic syndromes, ASD, and other psychiatric disorders), and psychosocial history. It is important to rule out other neurodevelopmental disorders including ID, specific learning disorders, stereotypic movement disorder, and tic disorders, which share some common clinical characteristics with ASD. It is also important to note that while many psychiatric disorders are associated with significant social impairment, the social deficits associated with ASD are unique in that they begin early in development, persist throughout life, and occur across multiple settings. Furthermore, the social impairment must be accompanied by restricted, repetitive patterns of behavior, which are unique to ASD and are rarely, if ever, seen in other disorders associated with social impairment.

All children who present with signs and symptoms concerning for ASD need to have a medical assessment, including a detailed physical examination, hearing screening, Wood's lamp examination for signs of tuberous sclerosis, and genetic testing. Initial genetic testing should include a G-banded karyotype, Fragile X syndrome testing, and a chromosomal microarray. Neuropsychological testing to assess for comorbid ID and learning disabilities, a speech and language evaluation to assess receptive and expressive language ability, and an occupational therapy (OT) evaluation to assess for sensory-motor deficits are also often recommended if there are developmental delays identified during the initial diagnostic assessment.

BIOLOGICAL TREATMENT

To date, no medication has been shown to consistently improve the core symptoms of ASD. Psychopharmacologic interventions may be a useful adjunct for the treatment of comorbid psychiatric disorders (e.g., ADHD, depression, anxiety, tics) or for behavioral symptoms associated with ASD like irritability (e.g., self-injury, physical aggression, severe tantrums) that interfere with the child's ability to access other nondrug therapeutic options. Pharmacologic treatments can be considered if the symptoms are severe or impairing, educational and behavioral interventions have been optimized, comorbid medical illness is ruled out, and psychosocial/environmental stressors are considered and addressed.

Risperidone and aripiprazole, both second-generation antipsychotics, are the only two medications approved by the Food and Drug Administration (FDA) for the treatment of irritability in children and adolescents with ASD. They have each been shown to be effective in reducing challenging behaviors associated with ASD but do not improve social functioning or language usage. The most common side effects associated with risperidone and aripiprazole are weight gain and sedation. With chronic use, these medications can also cause tardive dyskinesia. In addition to risperidone and aripiprazole, other first- and second-generation antipsychotics or mood stabilizers are sometimes used off-label to treat severe irritability in ASD. The need for the ongoing use of second-generation antipsychotics and/or mood stabilizers should be reassessed periodically and a gradual trial of tapering the medication may be warranted after a period of stability. Other psychotropic medications may be used off-label in ASD to treat commonly occurring comorbid psychiatric disorders such as ADHD, tics, anxiety disorders, sleep disorders, and mood disorders.

The principles for the psychopharmacologic management of individuals with ASD are the same as for individuals with other psychiatric conditions; however, it is important to keep in mind that children with ASD are generally more sensitive to medication side effects than typically developing children. Therefore, psychotropic agents should be started at lower doses and titrated more slowly in this population than in children without ASD.

PSYCHOSOCIAL TREATMENT

Intensive behavioral, developmental, and educational interventions are the primary components of treatment plans for ASD. Interventions for children with ASD should be multidimensional, multidisciplinary, and individualized according to the age and specific needs of the child. The goals of these interventions are to minimize core symptoms of ASD and associated behavioral problems while maximizing the individual's functional independence and overall quality of life by supporting the child to acquire adaptive skills. The American Academy of Child and Adolescent Psychiatry (AACAP) has published a Facts for Families document about ASD, which can be distributed to parents (https://www.aacap.org/AACAP/Families_and_Youth/Facts_for_Families/FFF-Guide/The-Child-With-Autism-011.aspx).

Educational Interventions

The Individuals with Disabilities Education Act (IDEA) is a law that guarantees a free and appropriate public education to eligible children with disabilities, including those with ASD (ages three to 21 years). Early intervention services under part C of IDEA covers the assessment of and intervention for children with developmental delays, including ASD, who are younger than three years of age. Once the child is eligible for school-based services, the public school system becomes responsible for providing services and education outlined in the Individualized Education Program (IEP), which is reviewed at least once a year. Some students who do not qualify for an IEP by educational criteria may be supported with accommodations through a Section 504 Plan or with classroom-level accommodations. Some children with ASD may need to be educated in special education classrooms or specialized schools for children with ASD. More specialized education settings can provide additional supports such as increased staffing, individual aides, or behavioral therapists.

Communication Interventions

Communication is a major focus of intervention and is typically addressed in the child's IEP in coordination with a speech and language pathologist. For individuals with fluent speech, the focus may be on pragmatic language skills training and the use of language in social contexts. This may include improving the child's ability to initiate conversation, respond to conversation, assess topic relevance, and use/assess nonverbal language such as eye contact and intonation. For children who are minimally verbal to nonverbal, augmentative and alternative communication (AAC) devices may be introduced. Optimizing a child with ASD's ability to communicate clearly and effectively is critical for improving quality of life and decreasing challenging behaviors.

Behavioral Interventions

Applied behavior analysis (ABA) is the most widely accepted evidence-based therapy for ASD. It uses principles of reinforcement to help children with ASD develop needed language, academic, and life skills, as well as decrease unwanted behaviors such as self-injury. Applied behavioral analysis teaches children skills in a stepwise progression and includes positive reinforcement.

Occupational Therapy

The goal of OT is to help children acquire the skills needed to perform the activities of daily living, improve gross and fine motor skills, modulate sensory processing, and enhance self-help skills.

KEY POINTS TO REMEMBER

- Autism spectrum disorder is a lifelong, highly heterogeneous neurodevelopmental disorder that requires a multidisciplinary, comprehensive treatment approach.
- There is no cure for ASD; however, early diagnosis and intervention have the potential to improve functional outcomes and quality of life.

- The treatment plan must be individualized based on the child's age and specific needs with the goals of maximizing functioning, moving the child toward independence, and improving quality of life.
- Pharmacologic treatment should be considered as one component of a broader, comprehensive multimodal treatment approach in the management of psychiatric comorbidities and maladaptive behaviors associated with ASD.

Further Reading

Hyman SL, Levy SE, Myers SM. Council on Children with Disabilities, Section on Developmental and Behavioral Pediatrics. Identification, evaluation, and management of children with autism spectrum disorder. *Pediatrics* 2020;145(1):e20193447.

Lord C, Elsabbagh M, Baird G, et al. Autism spectrum disorder. *Lancet* 2018;392(10146):508–520.

Palumbo ML, Keary CJ, McDougle CJ. Autism spectrum disorder (Chapter 7). In: McVoy M, Findling RL, eds. *Clinical Manual of Child and Adolescent Psychopharmacology*. 3rd ed. Washington, DC: American Psychiatric Publishing, 2017:307–359.

Volkmar F, Siegel M, Woodbury-Smith M, et al. Practice parameter for the assessment and treatment of children and adolescents with autism spectrum disorder. *J Am Acad Child Adolesc Psychiatry* 2014;53(2):237–257.

2 Persistent reading difficulty despite improved focus on a stimulant medication

Emily Anderberg

An eight-year-old girl with attention-deficit/hyperactivity disorder (ADHD) presents for an outpatient follow-up appointment. Her parents report that while her focus has improved on a stimulant medication, she is still struggling in most of her school subjects. In her third-grade class, she performs best on math assignments, though lately she has been struggling with word problems in math class. In early development she was slow to learn letters and their associated sounds. In her early school years, reading aloud seemed effortful and she sometimes guessed at entire words rather than sounding them out. She sometimes seems not to have understood what she has read. Her family history is significant for anxiety disorders and high school noncompletion.

Her school psychologist determined her intelligence quotient (IQ) is in the high average range. She showed a very low Overall Reading score (Standard Score = 68, second percentile), average Overall Mathematics score, and low average Overall Writing score with a weakness in spelling.

What Do You Do Now?

The patient has a specific learning disorder (SLD) with impairment in reading. This developmental disorder is characterized by difficulties learning a specific academic skill or skills, leading to substantially reduced achievement compared to same-age peers. For this patient, accessing specialized reading intervention as well as accommodations in school will be critical in helping her gain confidence, reduce stress, and learn efficiently in all her academic subjects.

EPIDEMIOLOGY

In the population of school-aged children, the prevalence of SLD is estimated to be 5% to 15%. The three subtypes of SLD are impairments in reading, written expression, and mathematics. Reading impairment is the most common subtype, occurring in about 80% of children with an SLD. About half of children with an SLD have more than one co-occurring subtype, with reading and writing as the most commonly codiagnosed areas of impairment. Specific learning disorder is about two to three times more common in boys than in girls. Risk factors include low birth weight, prenatal nicotine exposure, and family history (four to 10 times greater risk in those with first-degree relatives with SLD). About one-third of children with an SLD have comorbid ADHD.

SIGNS AND SYMPTOMS

According to the *Diagnostic and Statistical Manual of Mental Disorders*, Fifth Edition (DSM-5), an SLD is characterized by significant, persistent difficulties learning and using academic skills in one or more domains, despite the provision of interventions targeting the areas of deficit. Affected academic skills can include word reading, reading comprehension, spelling, written expression, number sense/calculation, and/or mathematical reasoning. The individual's specific academic skills must be quantifiably lower than their same-age peers (generally, 1.5 standard deviations below the mean, or below the seventh percentile), although low performance must not be attributable to more general concerns such as intellectual disability (ID), motor or sensory deficits, lack of educational opportunity, or low language proficiency. As SLD is a developmental disorder, the learning difficulties are present from the early school years but may not be detected until the academic demands exceed the student's skills.

The diagnosis of SLD must specify the affected academic skills, noting whether the individual displays impairment in reading, written expression, and/or mathematics. While not a DSM-specified subcategory, the term *dyslexia* refers to difficulties with fluent word reading, decoding, and spelling. Similarly, the term *dyscalculia* refers to difficulties learning arithmetic facts, processing numerical information, and performing fluent calculations. The term *dysgraphia* often refers to difficulties with both composition skills and handwriting.

ASSESSMENT

The diagnosis of an SLD requires a review of standardized academic achievement testing in combination with clinical interview and review of academic records. Cognitive testing may also be required to rule out ID and to provide a clearer picture of the child's learning needs. Academic achievement testing is often completed by a school psychologist or clinical psychologist. The most widely used tests to assess academic achievement include the Woodcock-Johnson Tests of Achievement and the Wechsler Individual Achievement Test, although other standardized measures have also been validated for this purpose. Providers reviewing achievement data should look for areas of distinct weakness falling 1.5 standard deviations below the mean, or below the seventh percentile. If achievement is globally reduced, other explanations besides SLD should be considered, such as ID, poor school attendance, low language proficiency in the language of instruction, severe anxiety, or another impairment (attention, motor, sensory, neurological) that would impact learning or performance. If there is substantial concern about low academic performance and standardized achievement testing has not been completed, the family can request testing through their school district's special education department or can be referred for neuropsychological testing.

Additionally, clinical interview and record review should include information about the student's classroom performance and what interventions the student has received to target areas of deficit (e.g., small group instruction, individual tutoring, extra work with parents). If the child has not received any interventions at home or at school, this must be attempted before the diagnosis is made, as remediation would indicate a delay or disruption in learning rather than a true learning disorder. Information about the progression of difficulties and early signs can distinguish SLD from a sudden onset of poor performance, which may be attributable to a change in psychosocial situation (e.g., trauma, life disruption) or neurological status. Providers should ask the child about their experiences with learning the subject and what they find difficult about the process. In combination with achievement testing, this information can provide clarity about the specific subtype of SLD and which interventions are needed. The clinical interview should also gauge the child's reaction to their difficulties, since anxiety disorders and major depressive disorder (MDD) are common among children and adolescents with an SLD. A family history of learning concerns (diagnosed or undiagnosed) can also provide data to support an SLD diagnosis.

BIOLOGICAL TREATMENT

There are no recognized or Food and Drug Administration (FDA)-approved medications for the treatment of SLD in either children or adults. Medications to support co-occurring psychiatric disorders (e.g., ADHD, MDD, or anxiety disorders) may provide an indirect benefit by helping the child better access instruction and other educational interventions.

PSYCHOSOCIAL TREATMENT

Experiencing learning difficulties can be very discouraging, and thus it is important for children and their families to receive psychoeducation about SLD. The American Psychiatric Association (APA) has published a helpful summary article on SLD (https://www.psychiatry.org/patients-families/specific-learning-disorder/what-is-specific-learning-disorder), which can be distributed to parents. Parents and providers can help children understand that they are not unintelligent or poor students, but rather their brains need to be taught in a different way. Children with SLD have higher-than-average rates of anxiety disorders, MDD, and suicidality, which may be responsive to psychotherapy.

Implementing appropriate educational interventions and accommodations as early as possible is critical to improving the child's performance and confidence. Students with an SLD are eligible for special education services under the Individuals with Disabilities Education Act (IDEA). The most effective interventions for SLD are generally individualized, intensive, and multimodal (e.g., multisensory). Services for students with an SLD in reading should be provided by a certified reading specialist. Students also benefit from accommodations in the classroom, such as extra time on testing, note-taking support, use of calculators, or verbally delivered instructions, depending on their specific needs. Medical providers can help families request an IEP evaluation and can support them in advocating for appropriate specialized interventions and accommodations.

KEY POINTS TO REMEMBER

- Specific learning disorder is a specific and substantial learning impairment that results in achievement scores below the seventh percentile.
- There are 5% to 15% of school-aged children who have an SLD, and many have more than one subtype.
- Specific learning disorder commonly co-occurs with ADHD and increases risk for anxiety disorders, MDD, and suicidality.
- Treatment includes specialized multimodal educational interventions in conjunction with academic accommodations.

Further Reading

Archibald LM, Cardy JO, Joanisse MF, et al. Language, reading, and math learning profiles in an epidemiological sample of school age children. *PloS One* 2013;8(10):e77463.

Hendren RL, Haft SL, Black JM, et al. Recognizing psychiatric comorbidity with reading disorders. *Front Psychiatry* 2018;9:101.

Lipkin PH, Okamoto J. The Individuals with Disabilities Education Act (IDEA) for children with special educational needs. *Pediatrics* 2015;136(6):e1650–e1662.

Pennington BF, McGrath LM, Peterson RL. *Diagnosing Learning Disorders: From Science to Practice.* 3rd ed. New York: Guilford Publications, 2019.

Voigt RG, Macias MM, Myers SM, Tapia CD, eds. *AAP Developmental and Behavioral Pediatrics.* 2nd ed. Itasca, IL: American Academy of Pediatrics, 2018.

3 Below-average intellectual and adaptive functioning

Cordelia Y. Ross

A nine-year-old boy is referred for the evaluation of aggressive behavior that has worsened over the past year. He experiences frequent outbursts of anger, screaming, and banging his head when upset. Sometimes he hits, bites, and kicks others who attempt to calm him. He has multiple developmental delays and requires assistance with bathing, eating, and dressing.

On psychiatric assessment, he exhibits limited eye contact and no spontaneous speech, but responds to questions with one- to two-word answers. He is hyperactive and engages in some repetitive behaviors such as hand flapping, excessive blinking, and occasional facial grimacing. Physical examination is notable for a long, narrow facies with large prominent ears, a high-arched palate, and hyperextendible finger joints. The remainder of his neurological exam is grossly normal.

What Do You Do Now?

The patient's presentation is suggestive of intellectual disability (ID) due to Fragile X syndrome (FXS), a genetic condition caused by a mutation of the *FMR1* gene on chromosome Xq27.3, leading to a range of developmental problems. Fragile X syndrome is the most common inherited cause of ID and is also associated with autism spectrum disorder (ASD) in approximately 50% of cases.

Intellectual disability is a neurodevelopmental disorder characterized by deficits in adaptive and intellectual functioning that begins during the developmental period. Intellectual disability replaces the older term "mental retardation" and has both syndromic and idiopathic etiologies. Global developmental delay describes those who have adaptive and intellectual difficulties before the age of five years when the clinical severity level cannot be reliably assessed during early childhood; some, but not all, of these children will go on to be diagnosed with ID.

With appropriate intervention and supports, many individuals with mild to moderate ID can live relatively independently with the appropriate supports and can engage in work. Life expectancy may be shortened, depending on the etiology of the disability. Some studies have shown that those with ID have an increased risk of developing dementia later in life, especially those with trisomy 21 (Down syndrome).

EPIDEMIOLOGY

Intellectual disability affects approximately 3% of the population in the United States, with severe ID affecting 1%. While ID is seen across socioeconomic groups, ethnicities, and educational levels, mild ID occurs more often in low socioeconomic groups, highlighting the correlation of intelligence quotient (IQ) with success in school and socioeconomic status. Intellectual disability is more common in boys, partially explained by X-linked causes of ID.

Etiologies of ID include genetic and environmental determinants and can be prenatal (e.g., congenital infections, prenatal drug or toxin exposure, severe undernutrition in pregnancy), perinatal (e.g., prematurity and other birth complications), or postnatal in origin (e.g., undernutrition and environmental deprivation during infancy and early childhood, viral and bacterial encephalitides and meningitides, severe head injury, asphyxia).

SIGNS AND SYMPTOMS

Children with ID may show abnormalities at birth or shortly thereafter, manifested by syndromic facial features or medical comorbidities suggesting developmental delay. Many children with ID, however, may not prompt concern until preschool, when parents and educators notice an inability to keep up with peers.

According to the *Diagnostic and Statistical Manual of Mental Disorders*, Fifth Edition (DSM-5), a diagnosis of ID is made by deficits in both adaptive and intellectual functioning, with difficulties presenting during the developmental period. Deficits in adaptive functioning highlight an inability to meet age- and socioculturally appropriate standards for independent functioning. Adaptive functioning deficits may be seen in three domains: conceptual (e.g., literacy [reading and writing], mathematics, self-direction, judgment in novel situations), social (e.g., interpersonal social communication, empathy, ability to relate to peers as friends, social problem solving), and practical (e.g., activities of daily living [eating, dressing, mobility, toileting], following a schedule or routine, occupational skills). Difficulties in intellectual function are defined as having an IQ of less than 70 (or greater than two standard deviations below the mean) with difficulty in reasoning, planning and problem solving, abstract thinking, and learning. Intelligence quotient ranges can help further classify the severity of ID into mild (IQ between 50 to 55 and 70), moderate (IQ between 35 to 40 and 50 to 55), severe (IQ between 20 to 25 and 35 to 40), and profound (IQ less than 20 to 25). The severity of ID should, however, ultimately be determined by the individual's functional abilities. In addition to determining ID severity, it is recommended that providers also assess the level of support a child may need in various activities of daily living.

ASSESSMENT

The assessment of ID involves screening for and evaluating underlying conditions associated with ID including genetic testing. Prenatal screening, such as ultrasonography, amniocentesis, chorionic villus sampling, and the quad screen test (alpha-fetoprotein, human chorionic gonadotropic, estriol, and inhibin A), may be done during pregnancy to identify conditions that often result in ID (e.g., trisomy 21, trisomy 18, or neural tube defects). Developmental screening during pediatrician well-child visits (e.g., Ages and Stages Questionnaires or Child Developmental Inventories) can quickly evaluate a child's cognitive, communicative, and motor skills and may prompt further, formal evaluation should a child fail to meet age-appropriate expectations. As discussed earlier, IQ testing may provide an indication of the severity of ID. The Stanford-Binet Intelligence Test and Wechsler Intelligence Scale for Children measure intellectual ability, while the Vineland Adaptive Behavior Scales, among other tests, can assess other areas of functioning, such as communication, daily living, social, and motor skills. Formal test results can provide evidence supporting a child's need for an Individualized Education Program (IEP) to access the educational curriculum (see more later under Psychosocial Treatment). Of note, children from diverse cultural backgrounds, non-English-speaking families, and families with very low socioeconomic status are more likely to do poorly on these tests; therefore, a diagnosis of ID requires a comprehensive clinical assessment that includes interviews with parents/caregivers and observation of the child, in addition to formal measures.

The evaluation of ID may also include a focused history and comprehensive physical examination; referral to a specialist (e.g., developmental pediatrician, pediatric neurologist, or psychologist); neurodevelopmental testing; school-based assessment; genetic evaluation; speech, language, and communication evaluation; vision and hearing screening; occupational and physical therapy assessment; and psychiatric referral for complex psychiatric needs (e.g., severe mood or behavioral problems). The need for additional evaluation with neuroimaging, electroencephalogram, genetic testing, and urine and blood tests depends on whether other aspects of the history and physical examination prompt further investigation.

There are several medical comorbidities associated with ID that may go under- or unrecognized and contribute to mood and/or behavioral changes. These include cerebral palsy, congenital heart disease, constipation, dental caries, endocrine abnormalities, gastroesophageal reflux disease, hearing loss, lead poisoning, obesity, seizures, sleep disorders, undescended testes, and vision impairment. Genetic disorders associated with ID include phenylketonuria, Tay-Sachs disease, FXS, Down syndrome, Prader-Willi syndrome, Angelman syndrome, Cornelia de Lange syndrome, Rett syndrome, and Williams syndrome, among many others.

Children with ID are at higher risk for comorbid psychiatric disorders than the general population. Psychiatric conditions associated with ID include anxiety disorders, ASD, attention-deficit/hyperactivity disorder (ADHD), major depressive disorder (MDD), dementia (early-onset), feeding/eating disorders, learning disorders, movement disorders, posttraumatic stress disorder, and self-injurious behaviors. Children who have been severely neglected and/or abused for prolonged periods of time may also present with signs and symptoms that mimic ID, highlighting the importance of a comprehensive evaluation.

BIOLOGICAL TREATMENT

There are no Food and Drug Administration (FDA)-approved medications for the treatment of ID; however, psychotropic medications may be used to manage mood or behavioral symptoms associated with psychiatric comorbidities. Antipsychotic medications can be used to treat agitation or irritability (aggression, self-injury, severe tantrums) refractory to behavioral strategies. Melatonin is often used as a first-line treatment for sleep difficulties. If MDD and/or an anxiety disorder are present and interfering, a selective serotonin reuptake inhibitor may be considered with close monitoring for side effects including behavioral activation. Stimulant and nonstimulant medications, such as alpha$_2$ adrenergic agonists or atomoxetine, may improve inattention and/or hyperactivity associated with co-occurring ADHD. Children with ID may be more sensitive to side effects of psychotropic medications. Therefore, medications should be started at the lowest possible dose and maintained at the lowest effective dosage to minimize the risk of side effects.

PSYCHOSOCIAL TREATMENT

The primary treatment of ID is identification and management of the associated medical and psychiatric conditions. Beyond this, goals of management are to decrease the effects of the disability by optimizing functioning at home, school, the community, and vocational settings. These may include helping the child to develop communication, adaptive living, and emotion regulation skills. Components of treatment may include speech and language therapy, occupational therapy, physical therapy, family counseling and respite care, behavioral interventions, educational assistance, case management, and assistive technology (for communication, mobility, etc.). When working with children with ID and their families, one is advised to communicate effectively (clearly, concisely, concretely), encourage independent functioning whenever possible, advocate for the child in their school and community, and collaborate with members of the child's team (e.g., educators, therapists, and other physicians).

Children with ID benefit from robust supports and services at home, at school, and in their communities. The Individuals with Disabilities Education Act (IDEA) provides early intervention and special education for children with disabilities from birth to age 21 years. Referrals should be made as soon as possible if a child has or is at risk for developing ID. Early intervention (ages three years and younger) includes a comprehensive evaluation and individualized multidisciplinary services, usually provided in the child's home. Special education (ages three to 21 years) provides school-based services with a focus on the least restrictive environment and may include accommodations according to Section 504 Plans and IEPs.

It is important to clarify issues of guardianship early on and make preparations for a child's transition to adulthood. Physicians are advised to address issues of sexuality, including options for birth control, principles of consent, and education regarding sexually transmitted infections. Furthermore, individuals with ID are at greatly increased risk for experiencing physical, sexual, or intimate partner violence; providers should screen for and remain vigilant about this. The American Academy of Child and Adolescent Psychiatry (AACAP) has published a Facts for Families article on ID, which can be distributed to parents (https://www.aacap.org/AACAP/Families_and_Youth/Facts_for_Families/FFF-Guide/Children-with-an-Intellectual-Disability-023.aspx#:~:text=Intellectual%20Disabilities&text=Intellectual%20disability%20(ID)%20is%20a,to%20function%20in%20everyday%20activities).

- Intellectual disability is characterized by deficits in intellectual and adaptive functioning beginning in childhood, and it affects 1% to 3% of the US population.
- Etiologies of ID include both genetic and environmental factors and can be prenatal, perinatal, and postnatal in origin.
- Management of ID consists of early detection, referral to early intervention and support services, investigation and treatment of any co-occurring illnesses (medical and/or psychiatric), and a comprehensive and team-based approach.
- Goals of intervention for children with ID are to minimize the effects of the disability and optimize functioning at home, at school, and in the community.

Further Reading

Michelson DJ, Shevell MI, Sherr EH, et al. Evidence report: Genetic and metabolic testing on children with global developmental delay: Report of the Quality Standards Subcommittee of the American Academy of Neurology and the Practice Committee of the Child Neurology Society. *Neurology* 2011;77(17):1629–1635.

Shevell M, Ashwal S, Donley D, et al. Practice parameter: Evaluation of the child with global developmental delay: Report of the Quality Standards Subcommittee of the American Academy of Neurology and The Practice Committee of the Child Neurology Society. *Neurology* 2003;60(3):367–380.

Sulkes SB. *Intellectual Disability, Professional Version*. Merck Manual. April 2020. Retrieved June 3, 2020, from https://www.merckmanuals.com/professional/pediatrics/learning-and-developmental-disorders/intellectual-disability#v1105033.

The Federation for Children with Special Needs and the Massachusetts Department of Education. *A Parent's Guide to Special Education*. Retrieved on 2020 June 3 from https://fcsn.org/parents-guide.

4 A child with inattention, hyperactivity, and impulsivity

Sirin Ozdemir and Craig L. Donnelly

Ryan is a seven-year-old boy presenting to his pediatrician due to behavioral dysregulation at school and at home. His teacher reports that Ryan seems unfocused, forgets to turn in assignments and struggles with completing tasks. He often blurts out answers, is "constantly running around" and has difficulty listening and following instructions. Ryan's mother reported he often complains of "stomachaches" before school and thinks his high level of anxiety is the cause of his behavior challenges. She feels his teacher should be doing more for his school-related anxiety. She insists on trying behavioral interventions before medication. Ryan was referred for anxiety-focused, group-based cognitive-behavioral therapy (CBT) after the initial assessment. The therapist noticed that Ryan seemed inattentive during group and could not finish the assigned tasks. He informed Ryan's parents that his anxiety was mostly performance related, owing to Ryan's inability to learn new information. He suggested they consider treating his "primary diagnosis" first, which may subsequently reduce anxiety symptoms.

What Do You Do Now?

The patient is suffering from attention-deficit/hyperactivity disorder (ADHD), a disorder that manifests in childhood with symptoms of inattention, hyperactivity, and impulsivity that occur in more than one setting and cause impairment in functioning. There are three presentations of ADHD: predominantly inattentive, predominantly hyperactive/impulsive, and combined. Each of these symptom domains may follow a different trajectory as the individual ages. Early identification and management of ADHD are important since it is one of the most common neurobehavioral disorders of childhood and causes significant impairment in a child's social, emotional, and academic development. Developing age-appropriate social skills and adequate peer functioning are also affected by ADHD. Hyperactivity and impulsivity may lead to peer rejection, and the overall negative consequences of social impairment may result in developing poor self-esteem and other psychiatric comorbidities (e.g., major depressive disorder [MDD], anxiety disorders, substance use disorders).

EPIDEMIOLOGY

According to the National Survey of Children's Health from 2016, 9.4% of children (14% in males and 6% in females) in the United States between the ages of two and 17 years have received an ADHD diagnosis. The male-to-female ratio is 4:1 for the predominantly hyperactive/impulsive presentation and is 2:1 for the predominantly inattentive presentation. Almost two-thirds of children with ADHD in this survey were taking medications for ADHD, approximately half had received behavioral treatment for ADHD, and almost one-fourth had received neither of these treatments. About half of children and adolescents with ADHD continue to exhibit impairing symptoms into adulthood. The prevalence of comorbid psychiatric disorders among children with ADHD ranges from 40% to 80% depending on the sample, with higher rates in clinically referred children (67% to 87%). Boys with ADHD are more likely to exhibit comorbid externalizing disorders (e.g., oppositional defiant disorder [ODD], conduct disorder [CD]), and girls are more likely to have internalizing disorders (e.g., anxiety disorders, MDD). Coexisting conditions may be either primary or exacerbated by ADHD, may affect the treatment response, and should be treated in conjunction with ADHD.

Although the etiology of ADHD remains unclear, emerging evidence suggests that it is related to a variety of factors including environmental, neurobiological, and genetic contributors. It is one of the most heritable psychiatric disorders and is associated with neurobiological deficits and dysregulation of the dopaminergic and noradrenergic systems. Etiologic studies have identified candidate genes including the dopamine (D4) receptor and the dopamine transporter, as well as certain prenatal and perinatal risk factors (e.g., smoking, viral infections, alcohol exposure, prematurity, low birth weight, and nutritional deficiency in the fetus).

SIGNS AND SYMPTOMS

According to the *Diagnostic and Statistical Manual of Mental Disorders*, Fifth Edition (DSM-5), ADHD is a childhood-onset disorder characterized by a persistent pattern of symptoms of developmentally inappropriate and impaired inattention, hyperactivity, and/or impulsivity. These symptoms should occur before the age of 12 years, last for at least six months, and be present in two or more settings (e.g., at home, school, or work; with friends; or in other activities). The DSM-5 includes specifiers to categorize ADHD based on subtype: predominantly inattentive, predominantly hyperactive-impulsive, and combined presentations. The subtype of ADHD may change during the course of an individual's development.

Six or more symptoms of hyperactivity-impulsivity need to be present for children and adolescents to meet DSM-5 criteria for hyperactivity/impulsivity. These include fidgetiness, difficulty remaining seated, running or climbing in inappropriate settings, inability to play or engage in leisure activities quietly, always being "on the go," talking excessively, blurting out answers before a question is completed, difficulty waiting their turn, and interrupting or intruding on others.

Six or more symptoms of inattention need to be present for children and adolescents to meet DSM-5 criteria for inattention. These include failure to provide close attention to detail and making careless mistakes; difficulty sustaining attention in activities; not seeming to listen when spoken to directly; failing to finish work; difficulty organizing tasks, activities, and belongings; avoiding tasks that require sustained mental effort; losing things necessary for tasks or activities; being forgetful; and being easily distracted by extraneous stimuli.

Hyperactive and impulsive symptoms are typically observed around age four years, peak in severity around seven to eight years, and then begin to decline. By adolescence, observable hyperactivity typically recedes; however, adolescents with ADHD may continue to feel internally restless. In contrast, the symptoms of inattention and impulsivity (e.g., substance abuse, risky sexual behavior, reckless driving) usually persist into adulthood.

ASSESSMENT

Children older than four years of age who present with symptoms of inattention, hyperactivity, or impulsivity should undergo an ADHD assessment based on interviews with the parent and patient, a comprehensive review of information about school functioning, screening for comorbid disorders, and developmental, medical, psychosocial, and family histories. The information required to diagnose ADHD should be obtained via standardized questionnaires and in-person discussions. Evaluation of the persistence and complications of the presenting symptoms while excluding differential diagnoses for the core symptoms and determining whether coexisting emotional, behavioral, and medical disorders are present is required to complete the assessment. Common disorders that coexist with ADHD include mood and anxiety disorders, specific learning disorders, language disorders, autism spectrum disorder, sleep disorders, tic disorders, substance use disorders, ODD, and CD. The examination should include observation for the presence of tics, as well as an assessment of the child's height, weight, pulse, and blood pressure.

The symptoms of ADHD overlap with a number of conditions including certain medical, developmental, neurologic, and psychiatric disorders, as well as psychosocial and environmental factors. A detailed medical history should be gathered including prenatal/perinatal complications, substance use, environmental exposures or infections, trauma, medical history, medications, and a family history. The review of systems should include information about sleep impairment, cardiac history, and nutrition before considering medication trials to avoid attributing pre-existing symptoms to medication-related adverse effects. Environmental exposures (e.g., lead, tobacco), trauma (e.g., neglect, abuse), family stress, risk of medication misuse by the child or family members, and educational history are important aspects of the psychosocial history.

It is not uncommon for children with ADHD to deny or be unaware of their symptoms. Therefore, either observing the child in the school setting or collecting information from parents and teachers is critical for making the diagnosis. Rating scales should be completed by both the child's parents and teachers to collect structured observations of the child's behavior and determine whether ADHD symptoms occur in more than one setting. Clinician-administered ADHD rating scales have a sensitivity and specificity of greater than 90%. The Vanderbilt Assessment Scales can be downloaded and printed from the National Initiative for Children's Healthcare Quality (NICHQ) website (https://www.nichq.org/sites/default/files/resource-file/NICHQ_Vanderbilt_Assessment_Scales.pdf).

BIOLOGICAL TREATMENT

Medications for ADHD are divided into two major categories: stimulant and nonstimulant medications. Stimulants are further divided into two categories: methylphenidates and amphetamines (dextroamphetamine and mixed dextroamphetamine-amphetamine salts). Stimulants promote the release of dopamine and norepinephrine from presynaptic nerve terminals and block the reuptake of these catecholamines by competitive inhibition. They are the first-line medication class for the treatment of ADHD. A variety of stimulant formulations are available in immediate-, extended-, and sustained-release preparations as well as liquid, chewable, and sprinkle forms. Sustained-release preparations offer several advantages including once-daily dosing, decreased potential for misuse, and continuous coverage of ADHD symptoms throughout the day. Stimulants are effective in the majority of patients (about 70%) and are generally considered to be safe. Most of their side effects are mild, short in duration, and reversible. The most common side effects of stimulants include appetite suppression, abdominal pain, headaches, sleep impairment, jitteriness, and emotional lability. Less common side effects include poor growth or weight loss and increased blood pressure. Psychosis (hallucinations) is a very rare but serious side effect. There have been historical concerns about sudden cardiac death and new-onset tic disorders among children treated with stimulants; however, the evidence does not support either of these concerns. Recent studies also show that the use of stimulant medications is safe in children with epilepsy if they are appropriately treated with anticonvulsants. Finally, parents and providers may hesitate to use stimulant medications because they are classified as controlled substances. While ADHD in and of itself is associated with an increased risk of substance misuse, it is important to note that the evidence suggests an overall decreased lifetime risk of developing substance use disorders if ADHD symptoms are treated with stimulant medications.

Nonstimulant medications for the treatment of ADHD include a selective norepinephrine reuptake inhibitor (atomoxetine) and two selective alpha$_2$ adrenergic agonists (guanfacine and clonidine). They can reduce the core symptoms of ADHD but are not as effective as stimulants. Therefore, nonstimulant medications should be considered if there are concerns about the misuse of stimulants or if intolerable side effects from stimulants occur. The alpha$_2$ adrenergic agonists may be particularly helpful if the patient has a comorbid tic disorder. Common side effects of atomoxetine include somnolence, appetite suppression, and gastrointestinal symptoms (particularly with rapid dose increase). Increased suicidal thoughts, sudden death in children with pre-existing serious cardiac problems, and hepatitis are rare but serious side effects. Similar to antidepressants, atomoxetine carries a Food and Drug Administration (FDA) black box warning of increased suicidality in children and adolescents. The most common side effects of alpha$_2$ adrenergic agonists include somnolence, dry mouth, and hypotension. They must be tapered gradually to avoid rebound hypertension.

Medications, particularly stimulants, with or without behavioral/ psychologic interventions are considered the mainstay of treatment for ADHD in children and adolescents six years and older.

There is no FDA-approved medication for the treatment of ADHD in preschool-aged children (four to five years). Furthermore, stimulants have been shown to be both less well tolerated and less effective in younger children. Behavioral interventions should be tried first in this age group. If symptoms do not respond to or interfere with behavioral interventions or cause safety concerns or loss of educational opportunities (e.g., exclusion from preschool/daycare), medications may be considered in addition to behavioral therapy. Methylphenidates should be considered before using the amphetamine class of stimulants or nonstimulant medications, since most of the evidence for the safety and efficacy of treating preschool children has been from methylphenidates.

PSYCHOSOCIAL TREATMENT

Psychoeducation and school-based interventions are important components of the treatment plan for ADHD. The American Academy of Child and Adolescent Psychiatry (AACAP) has published a Facts for Families guide on ADHD, which can be distributed to parents (https://www.aacap.org/AACAP/Families_and_Youth/Facts_for_Families/FFF-Guide/Children-Who-Cant-Pay-Attention-Attention-Deficit-Hyperactivity-Disorder-006.aspx). Psychoeducation should include educating the child's parents about the disorder and teaching them how to help manage the child's environment to decrease extraneous distraction and aid in providing consistency.

Ensuring an appropriate educational environment is another important component of treatment. Classroom modifications that can be helpful for children and adolescents with ADHD include preferential seating near the teacher, organizational tools (e.g., homework notebook, schedule), a consistent classroom routine, a plan for how the teacher can cue the child without drawing negative attention, and allowing the child to take frequent movement breaks. If these types of modifications are insufficient, children with ADHD may qualify for special education under the Individuals with Disabilities Education Act (IDEA) or for more intensive accommodations within the regular classroom setting under Section 504 of the Rehabilitation Act of 1973. The need for special education services should be determined after the maximum benefit from medication treatments has been achieved. Special education services for ADHD may include smaller classroom size, access to a resource room, one-to-one tutoring, or a more intensive out-of-district special education placement.

Unlike most other psychiatric disorders, there is strong evidence for medication-only treatment without therapy as being the most efficacious intervention for ADHD. The Multimodal Treatment Study of Children with ADHD (MTA) study demonstrated that the combination of behavioral therapy and stimulant medication was not superior to stimulant medication-only treatment of ADHD. However, patients with coexisting disorders and/or psychosocial stressors had benefit from adjunctive psychosocial interventions (particularly those with comorbid anxiety disorders, ODD, and CD). Therefore, psychosocial treatment can be considered in combination with medications for the treatment of ADHD if a patient has a partial response to medications, has a coexisting psychiatric disorder, or is experiencing psychosocial stressors. Adjunctive psychotherapy treatments that may benefit some children and adolescents with ADHD include social skills training and cognitive behavioral therapy that focuses on executive functioning, problem solving, and organization.

KEY POINTS TO REMEMBER

- Attention-deficit/hyperactivity disorder is one of the most common neuropsychiatric disorders of childhood and often persists into adulthood.
- Treatment of ADHD may involve behavioral/psychologic interventions, medication, and/or educational interventions, alone or in combination. The first-line treatment approach varies with the age of the child.
- Stimulants are highly effective and safe when used appropriately.
- Behavioral interventions should be considered as the initial treatment for preschool-aged children with ADHD.
- Medication treatment should be considered first line for school-aged children and adolescents.
- Behavioral/psychotherapeutic interventions may not provide benefit for core symptoms of ADHD but may reduce symptoms of coexisting comorbidities.

Further Reading

Pliszka S; AACAP Work Group on Quality Issues. Practice parameter for the assessment and treatment of children and adolescents with attention-deficit/hyperactivity disorder. *J Am Acad Child Adolesc Psychiatry* 2007;46(7):894–921.

Wolraich ML, Hagan JF Jr, Allan C, et al. Clinical practice guideline for the diagnosis, evaluation, and treatment of attention-deficit/hyperactivity disorder in children and adolescents [published correction appears in *Pediatrics*. 2020 Mar;145(3):e20193997]. *Pediatrics* 2019;144(4):e20192528.

Molina BS, Hinshaw SP, Swanson JM, et al. The MTA at 8 years: Prospective follow-up of children treated for combined-type ADHD in a multisite study. *J Am Acad Child Adolesc Psychiatry* 2009;48:484–500.

5 Repetitive throat clearing, blinking, and grimacing

Danielle Sipsock

A nine-year-old boy presents to his psychiatrist where he is being treated for worries centered around social interactions with peers. His mother reports he has been increasingly anxious about going to school.

On assessment, the boy appears nervous and clears his throat repeatedly. He states he hates going to school due to his peers teasing him about facial movements that have worsened over the past three weeks. They bully him about blinking his eyes frequently and a facial grimace that he cannot control. He has had these movements for the past three years, but they have worsened recently. Both of these movements are present during the interview. They are nonrhythmic, rapid movements. He states these movements are involuntary, but he can suppress them for a short period of time. Some days the movements are worse than others. He worries about what others think of him and tries to avoid being called on in class, which is affecting his school performance.

What Do You Do Now?

The diagnosis for this patient is Tourette's disorder, given the presence of multiple motor and vocal tics. According to the *Diagnostic and Statistical Manual of Mental Disorders*, Fifth Edition (DSM-5), a tic is a sudden, rapid, recurrent, nonrhythmic motor movement or vocalization and can be simple or complex. Simple tics are sudden, brief, repetitive movements that involve a limited number of muscle groups, while complex tics are coordinated patterns of movements involving several muscle groups. Tic disorders are especially important for psychiatrists to identify in their patients as they may lead to functional impairment or increase risk for depressive symptoms and/or stress due to peer difficulties.

EPIDEMIOLOGY

Tics are very common in school-aged children, with a large, community-based study demonstrating that more than 19% of school-aged children have had at least one type of tic. Tic disorders occur in about 1% of the population. Importantly, tics and tic disorders are three to four times more common in boys than in girls. Tourette's disorder, defined as the presence of multiple motor tics and at least one vocal tic where tics persist for at least one year, is estimated to affect 0.3% to 1% of the population. Although possible environmental and prenatal influences are under investigation, the main known risk factor is the presence of a tic disorder in a first-degree relative. Motor tics typically appear between the ages of four and six years, with vocal tics appearing a few years later. Simple tics typically precede complex tics. Tic disorders peak in prevalence and severity around age nine to 14 years before diminishing, with the majority (65%) of individuals spontaneously achieving remission by late adolescence/early adulthood. When tics first appear, it is difficult to determine whether they will follow a self-remitting or a chronic course. A particular tic can recur over a period of days, weeks, or months. It is then usually either followed by a period of waning or replaced by another tic. With age, tics can worsen in frequency and severity, peaking during early adolescence. Studies indicate that around 75% of people who present with a tic disorder before the age of 10 years have a significant decrease in symptoms during adolescence, while the remaining 25% have persisting or worsening of symptoms into adulthood. Although childhood tics do not predict long-term outcomes, tics are often comorbid with other psychiatric disorders, most commonly attention-deficit/hyperactivity disorder (ADHD) and obsessive-compulsive disorder (OCD), which in and of themselves are associated with poorer functioning.

SIGNS AND SYMPTOMS

Tic disorders are categorized as neurodevelopmental disorders in the DSM-5. This category encompasses multiple disorders that are hierarchical in order of severity and persistence: Tourette's disorder, persistent (chronic) motor or vocal tic disorder, provisional tic disorder, other specified tic disorder, and unspecified tic disorder. Once a tic disorder diagnosis at one level of the hierarchy is made, a lower-hierarchy diagnosis cannot be made. To meet criteria for Tourette's disorder, persistent motor or vocal tic disorder, and provisional tic disorder, the patient must have the onset of tics before 18 years of age and tics cannot be attributable to a medical condition or physiologic effect of a substance. If tics have been present for less than one year since any tic first appeared, then the diagnosis is provisional tic disorder. If tics have been present for more than one year, then Tourette's disorder and persistent motor or vocal tic disorder are used. Tourette's disorder requires multiple motor and one or more vocal tics, while persistent motor or vocal tic disorder requires that single or multiple motor OR vocal tics have been present, but not both. Persistent motor or vocal tic disorder thus requires specifiers of either "motor tics only" or "vocal tics only." Other specified and unspecified tic disorders are used in presentations where symptoms characteristic of a tic disorder cause significant distress or impairment but do not meet full criteria for the aforementioned tic disorders or any other specific neurodevelopmental disorder, such as tic disorders presenting after the age of 18 years.

Tics typically wax and wane in severity over time and can worsen with stress or strong emotions. They may present in various combinations, which can also change over time. Simple motor tics can include eye blinking, facial grimacing, shoulder jerks, or head jerking. Simple vocal tics can include repetitive throat clearing, sniffing, or grunting sounds. Complex motor tics may be more difficult to identify. Complex motor tics may appear purposeful, such as hopping, foot tapping, or twisting. Complex vocal tics may include repeated words or phrases that appear to be out of context.

ASSESSMENT

It is recommended that tic disorders be screened for in every psychiatric interview, given the high comorbidity with other psychiatric disorders and their potential effect on functioning. Questions should be asked about any abnormal or unwanted repetitive movements or vocalizations. Many families or patients attribute common tics such as sniffing, coughing, or blinking to allergies or vision changes. If a screen is positive for tics, a comprehensive assessment of these symptoms is warranted.

A comprehensive tic evaluation should include a discussion of the reported movements and/or vocalizations and probing for additional ones. The characteristics of and a timeframe for each tic should be established. Additional clinical features to assess include severity, frequency, triggers, alleviating factors, accompanying sensations, the patient's ability to suppress the movement, and whether there is a premonitory urge. These features can help establish or differentiate tic disorders from other conditions. Tics are differentiated from most other movement disorders by the ability of the patient to temporarily suppress tics, the patient's perception that a tic relieves some type of inner tension, and a preceding premonitory urge. When tics are suppressed, the individual experiences a buildup of inner tension until the tic is expressed. Tics are often preceded by a premonitory urge, resembling the need to sneeze. Intense concentration also suppresses tics. Caregivers and patients should be asked how the tics are problematic to evaluate potential functional impairment. If the diagnosis is not clear after a thorough assessment, rating scales may be helpful. The Yale Global Tic Severity Scale (YGTSS) is a clinician-administered tool noted in the field to be one of the most comprehensive, valid, and reliable. The Tourette's Disorder Scale (TODS) is a shorter tool that can also be useful and is available as a parent or clinician rating scale. Patients being assessed for tic disorders should also have a psychiatric assessment for co-occurring psychiatric conditions (e.g., ADHD and OCD), as they are very common and may impact treatment choices.

An initial evaluation of tics should also include a developmental/birth history, medication history, family history (neurologic and psychiatric), and assessment of family dynamics and functioning. Although tic disorders may be idiopathic, they can also be the result of medications or general medical conditions. It has been a longstanding worry of many families that stimulant medications, including methylphenidate and amphetamine-related compounds, cause or increase tics, which controlled studies have not supported despite Food and Drug Administration (FDA) inserts listing tics as a potential side effect. Other psychiatric medications such as selective serotonin reuptake inhibitors (SSRIs) or lamotrigine have also been reported to increase or unmask tics. Recreational use of certain substances, such as amphetamines, methamphetamines, or cocaine, can also increase or unmask tics. Other than medication- or substance-induced tics, the differential diagnosis can include a variety of movement disorders and neurologic diseases such as stereotypies, seizures, and dystonias. For this reason, a neurologic examination or neurology referral may be warranted to ensure an accurate diagnosis, particularly in the context of declining cognitive or motor function. A medical workup should be considered for new-onset tics and may include complete blood count, complete metabolic panel including hepatic function tests, thyroid function tests, ferritin, or urine drug screen. For sudden symptom onset or those with other neurologic findings, indicated labs may include a workup for viral illness or brain imaging, in which case a consultation with a pediatric specialist most likely would also be indicated.

BIOLOGICAL TREATMENT

Biological treatments for tic disorders center around psychopharmacologic interventions. It is important to note that medications may not be first line for the treatment of tics, and "watchful waiting" or starting with psychosocial treatments may be preferable. Since tic symptoms often do not cause impairment, the majority of children meeting criteria for tic disorders do not require medications for tic suppression. For all of the medications discussed next, the risks of side effects should always be balanced with the reported level of impairment by the patient and caregiver. Most parameters recommend initiation of medication treatment only if tics are moderate to severe and causing severe impairment, or if psychiatric conditions are co-occurring and a medication may target both disorders. The goal of treatment, which should be conveyed to patients and their families, is symptom reduction, not remission. Thus, medications should be titrated to the lowest effective dose that addresses functional impairment.

Medications with FDA approval for the treatment of Tourette's disorder include haloperidol, pimozide, and aripiprazole. Clinicians often prefer using second-generation antipsychotics (especially aripiprazole and risperidone) given their different side effect profile from first-generation antipsychotics. Lower doses of these medications are indicated for tic disorders than for mood or psychotic disorders. Common side effects within these drug classes depend on the medication but commonly include weight gain, sedation, QTc interval prolongation, and extrapyramidal symptoms. If stopped, these medications should be tapered over weeks to months to minimize withdrawal dyskinesias.

Despite not having FDA approval for treatment of tic disorders, many clinicians prefer the initial use of alpha$_2$ adrenergic agonists for tic suppression, given their safer side effect profile. Both clonidine and guanfacine are used, with clonidine thought to be more likely to reduce tic severity and both having improved efficacy when treating tics that are comorbid with ADHD. Common side effects include sedation, drowsiness, hypotension, bradycardia, and rebound hypertension with abrupt discontinuation.

Other medications with lower levels of evidence for treating tics are SSRIs, particularly when the patient also has OCD, and treatment of localized and bothersome simple motor tics in adolescents and adults with botulinum toxin injections. Deep brain stimulation and repetitive transcranial magnetic stimulation are being investigated as potential treatments, but at this time the American Academy of Child and Adolescent Psychiatry (AACAP) practice parameters do not recommend neurostimulation for the treatment of tic disorders.

Determining how to decide when to stop a medication that is treating tics should be done collaboratively with the patient, caregiver, and physician. It is important to remember that the natural course of tics is typically to improve throughout adolescence and early adulthood. Thus, medications may be able to be reduced or stopped, with either decreased or resolved tics. Families may also choose to lower or stop medications during the summer or other times when there is less stress and symptoms are less interfering.

PSYCHOSOCIAL TREATMENT

After a tic disorder has been established, psychoeducation should be provided to the family and patient including the prevalence, symptoms, typical course, and management options. The Facts for Families article about Tic disorders published by the AACAP can be used to support this discussion (https://www.aacap.org/App_Themes/AACAP/docs/facts_for_families/ 35_tic_disorders.pdf).

Families should be made aware of local and national advocacy groups such as the Tourette Association of America that provide resources and support. Advocacy groups publish a wealth of information targeted toward youth, educators, and parents including about school-based modifications. Recommendations for the school can be very helpful, including providing teachers destigmatizing education about tics and acquiring educational accommodations through an Individual Education Program (IEP) or 504 Plan. Educational accommodations may include items such as the teacher ignoring tics or the patient's ability to leave the classroom. Psychoeducation targeted to teachers and peers may also be beneficial, and the Tourette Association of America and Home Box Office (HBO) produced a film and teacher's guide to facilitate this (https://tourette.org/about-tourette/ tourettes-doesnt-have-me/).

The first-line behavioral intervention for tic disorders is habit reversal training (HRT); comprehensive behavioral intervention for tics (CBIT) is a well-known and utilized variant. Habit reversal training involves an intervention to eliminate the premonitory urge of a tic and is supported by randomized controlled trials for moderate to severe tic disorders. Therapist and parent handbooks are both available. There is some preliminary evidence that HRT may be delivered through telemedicine rather than in person and still be an effective treatment. Although in initial studies HRT compared favorably to placebo, a recent study has demonstrated that HRT is as equally efficacious at improving quality of life and reducing tic severity as antipsychotic medications. Second-line psychotherapies include exposure and response prevention, which is a form of cognitive behavioral therapy, and skill-based therapies that target distortions/avoidance around tics and aim to improve adaptive coping mechanisms.

- Tic disorders peak in late childhood and commonly co-occur with other psychiatric disorders.
- Tics are sudden, rapid, recurrent, nonrhythmic motor movements or vocalizations and can be simple or complex.
- Assessment should include ruling out nonidiopathic causes of tics including medications, substance use, and general medical conditions such as neurologic and movement disorders.
- Treatment should start with psychoeducation and focus on symptom reduction rather than remission with the goal of maximizing functioning and quality of life.
- Behavioral interventions, particularly HRT, should be considered if tics cause impairment and are moderate in severity OR are present with psychiatric comorbidities that may be responsive to the proposed behavioral treatment.
- Medications, such as antipsychotics and alpha$_2$ adrenergic agonists, should be considered if tics cause severe impairment and are moderate to severe OR are present with psychiatric comorbidities that may be responsive to the proposed medication.

Further Reading

Cath DC, Hedderly T, Ludolph AG, et al. European clinical guidelines for Tourette syndrome and other tic disorders. Part I: Assessment. *Eur Child Adolesc Psychiatry* 2011;20(4):155–171.

Essoe JK, Grados MA, Singer HS, et al. Evidence-based treatment of Tourette's disorder and chronic tic disorders. *Expert Rev Neurother* 2019;19(11):1103–1115.

Murphy TK, Lewin AB, Storch EA, et al. Practice parameter for the assessment and treatment of children and adolescents with tic disorders. *J Am Acad Child Adolesc Psychiatry* 2013;52(12):1341–1359.

Pringsheim T, Okun MS, Müller-Vahl K, et al. Practice guideline recommendations summary: Treatment of tics in people with Tourette syndrome and chronic tic disorders. *Neurology* 2019;92(19):896–906.

Rizzo R, Pellico A, Silvestri PR, et al. A randomized controlled trial comparing behavioral, educational, and pharmacological treatments in youths with chronic tic disorder or Tourette syndrome. *Front Psychiatry* 2018;9:100.

Walkup JT, Mink JW, McNaught K, eds. *A Family's guide to Tourette Syndrome.* Bloomington, IN: iUniverse, 2012.

6 Teenager with paranoia and hallucinations preceded by a decline in academic and social functioning

Joseph A. Pereira

A 17-year-old boy is seen with his parents in the emergency department for "unusual behavior" including talking about conspiracy theories and concerns that the government is spying on him. The prior night, he boarded up his windows because he was afraid others were watching him. He previously was an average student with three to four close friends. However, about one year ago, he began spending less time with others and now rarely leaves his room.

On psychiatric assessment, he appears to be responding to an auditory stimulus not heard by others. When asked about the voices, he responds: "I can't tell you. You are not to be trusted." His mother notes he has no prior psychiatric conditions but did receive a few counseling sessions from his pediatrician's office on marijuana use about two years ago. His mother reports that he has not been using any substances recently and his urine toxicology screen in the emergency department is negative.

What Do You Do Now?

This adolescent is exhibiting symptoms of schizophrenia, a primary psychotic disorder that results from interactions between genetic, environmental, and neurobiological factors. Schizophrenia is a chronic condition, associated with significant impairments in social, educational, and occupational functioning as well as early mortality. Childhood-onset schizophrenia (COS), defined by a first appearance of symptoms before the age of 13 years, is very rare, while early-onset schizophrenia (EOS), characterized by an initial symptom presentation between the ages of 14 and 18 years, is more common. Early recognition, diagnosis, and treatment are imperative, as untreated schizophrenia, specifically the duration of untreated psychosis, is associated with poor outcomes.

EPIDEMIOLOGY

The symptoms of schizophrenia typically begin between the ages of 15 and 30 years. The lifetime prevalence of schizophrenia among adults is approximately 1%. Childhood-onset schizophrenia is exceedingly rare, with a prevalence of one to two per 100,000 children, with a male predominance. The prevalence of schizophrenia increases rapidly after the age of 14 years, particularly in males. Early-onset schizophrenia is much less rare than COS, making up a total of approximately 30% of all cases of schizophrenia. Compared with adult-onset schizophrenia, COS and EOS are associated with poorer prognosis including more severe illness, lower premorbid functioning, and more severe negative symptoms (e.g., anhedonia, affective flattening, anergy, apathy, paucity of speech, and cognitive slowing). Thirty percent of individuals with EOS will require long-term intensive supports for daily functioning. Schizophrenia symptom onset is often insidious in children and adolescents, marked by a deterioration of or failure to meet expected social or academic levels of achievement. A family history of schizophrenia is the most significant risk factor for developing schizophrenia. Individuals with a first-degree relative with schizophrenia are at 10 times increased risk of developing schizophrenia than the general population. Other risk factors for schizophrenia include a history of obstetrical complications; premorbid social, motor, and language impairments; academic decline; marijuana use; structural neurobiological defects (e.g., increased lateral ventricle volumes on magnetic resonance imaging scans); residence in an urban environment; history of migration, both international and within-country; and ethnic minority identity. Psychosocial factors, such as high "expressed emotion" in families, do not cause the disorder but may influence its severity and rate of recurrence. Suicidality is a common comorbid feature, with at least 5% of individuals with EOS dying by suicide or accidental death related to their psychosis. Good prognostic indicators of schizophrenia include shorter duration of untreated psychosis, fewer negative symptoms, predominantly only delusions and hallucinations as positive symptoms (disorganized behavior and disorganized speech are poor prognostic indicators), higher premorbid baseline functioning, and onset associated with an acute precipitating stressor.

SIGNS AND SYMPTOMS

According to the *Diagnostic and Statistical Manual of Mental Disorders*, Fifth Edition (DSM-5), two or more of the following symptoms must be present to make the diagnosis of schizophrenia: hallucinations, delusions, disorganized speech, disorganized or catatonic behavior, and/or negative symptoms. At least one of the symptoms must be hallucinations, delusions, or disorganized speech. There must be an associated decline in functioning, which is most notable in the domains of academic and social functioning in youth. There must be continuous signs of the disturbance for at least six months, with at least one month of active symptoms, although this duration may be shortened with the appropriate treatment. The DSM-5 specifiers can be used to characterize the course of the disorder (first vs. multiple episodes; acute episode vs. partial remission vs. full remission), whether catatonia is present, and the current severity.

The symptoms of schizophrenia can be separated into two categories: positive and negative symptoms. Positive symptoms refer to the presence of hallucinations, delusions, disorganized speech, and disorganized behavior. Psychosis, which collectively refers to hallucinations and delusions, is defined generally as a disturbance in thought and/or behavior that leads to impaired reality testing. Negative symptoms refer to deficits, such as anhedonia, affective flattening, anergy, apathy, paucity of speech, and cognitive slowing.

There are generally four phases of schizophrenia: the prodromal phase (marked by a decline in functioning), the acute phase (characterized by pronounced positive symptoms), the recuperative/recovery phase (several-month period with remission of active symptoms, continued impairment, and significant negative symptoms), and the residual phase (extended phase without positive symptoms, with some impairment still noticeable).

Early-onset schizophrenia is considered to be the same disorder as adult-onset schizophrenia and is diagnosed using the same criteria. Delusions and catatonic symptoms are known to occur less frequently in those diagnosed before the age of 18 years, while cognitive deficits are seen more commonly in EOS. The most common symptoms of EOS include hallucinations, thought disorder, and flattened affect.

ASSESSMENT

The assessment of a child or adolescent with a suspected diagnosis of schizophrenia requires integrated biological, psychological, and social approaches. Currently, the psychiatric interview remains the gold standard for establishing the diagnosis. Inquiry into the child's symptomatology should include the child, the child's caregiver(s), and other informants such as teachers or coaches. Children and adolescents with schizophrenia are typically able to describe their psychotic symptoms when prompted, but accurate reporting can be hindered by active paranoia or disorganization. Younger children may be more easily engaged using play-based interview techniques. Because of these factors, caregivers, teachers, and other individuals who are close to the individual can provide invaluable information about how the child's behavior, functioning, and thinking have changed.

A developmental approach should be taken when assessing a child's symptoms using the DSM-5 criteria. Many children have intense imaginations that can be misinterpreted as psychosis, despite being developmentally typical. In addition, developmental disorders can present with language and cognitive impairments that can make it difficult to differentiate them from schizophrenia.

It is critical to evaluate the longitudinal pattern of a child's symptoms in conjunction with the mental status examination to improve the accuracy of the diagnosis. While the exact features of a mental status examination can vary, individuals with schizophrenia may appear unkempt, have a restricted affect, report seeing or hearing things that are not perceived by the examiner, and express bizarre and unrealistic delusions. Speech may be characterized by long pauses before answering questions, a consequence of thought blocking, while thought processes may be illogical, with a circumstantial stream and looseness of associations.

Biological Assessment

A complete medical history and physical examination including neurological evaluation are required to rule out the possibility of medical conditions that might lead to the development of psychotic symptoms, such as drug intoxication or withdrawal, medication side effects (e.g., stimulants or corticosteroids), or other medical conditions. Medical conditions that can cause psychotic symptoms include central nervous system disorders (e.g., viral encephalitis, intracranial neoplasms, head trauma, congenital malformation, seizure disorder), toxic exposures (e.g., carbon monoxide, heavy metals), and rheumatologic disorders (e.g., systemic lupus erythematous). Baseline routine laboratory tests, including toxicology screening, complete blood count, serum electrolytes, liver enzymes, renal function, thyroid-stimulating hormone, folate, and vitamin B12, should be obtained. Additional tests such as for hepatitis C, syphilis, Wilson's disease, and rheumatologic causes may also be considered based on the clinical presentation and physical examination findings. A formal neurological consultation should be considered if the history and/or physical examination suggest an underlying neurologic etiology. Neuroimaging is no longer routinely recommended in first-episode psychoses in the absence of signs or symptoms of intracranial pathology due to the risks of radiation exposure and delayed treatment. Signs and symptoms suggestive of intracranial pathology include focal neurologic signs, headaches, nausea and vomiting, and seizure-like activity.

Psychological Assessment

There is no psychological test that can establish the diagnosis of schizophrenia; however, neuropsychological testing early during the course of schizophrenia is recommended to document baseline cognitive functioning as well as to guide therapeutic and academic interventions. Baseline and follow-up rating scales such as the Positive and Negative Syndrome Scale (PANSS) and the Symptom Onset in Schizophrenia (SOS) can be helpful to establish the severity of baseline symptoms and determine the response to treatment. Trauma and neglect history should be ascertained and evaluated in the context of the child's presentation. Inquiry into premorbid and co-morbid behavioral challenges, cognitive delays, learning difficulties, and social isolation should also be completed.

Social Assessment

Individuals with schizophrenia often present with social difficulties and a lack of interest in relationships. Social impairment is seen throughout each phase of the illness and can begin even prior to the prodromal phase. Compromised social functioning portends a poor clinical outcome and thus necessitates early recognition and intervention. Signs of impaired social functioning in individuals often include impaired relatedness, poor hygiene, and confrontations with peers.

There are several cultural factors that can influence the presentation and assessment of schizophrenia. In particular, migration status (particularly first- and second-generation immigrants) and residence in an urban environment are associated with higher rates of schizophrenia. In addition, as cultural, religious, and societal norms can interface with both the presentation and interpretation of psychotic symptoms, it is important to differentiate between true psychosis and culturally accepted beliefs.

Differential Diagnosis

Several psychiatric conditions can present with features similar to schizophrenia, including depression with psychotic features, schizoaffective disorder, posttraumatic stress disorder, bipolar disorder, personality disorders, and developmental disorders. Some features of autism spectrum disorder, such as concrete thinking, social withdrawal, and inappropriate affect, may also resemble features of schizophrenia. Several medical conditions can also mimic characteristics of schizophrenia, particularly positive symptoms. Particular attention to the mental status examination and adherence to the DSM-5 diagnostic criteria can aid in arriving at the correct diagnosis. Importantly, features of schizophrenia that are relatively unique to this diagnosis include insidious onset of symptoms accompanied by clear functional decline usually during adolescence, retrospective history of a prodromal period, and at least two positive symptoms (one of which must be hallucinations, delusions, or disorganized speech) that are sustained over several months.

Schizophrenia is highly comorbid with several conditions. It is imperative to conduct regular safety assessments, as suicidal ideation is common. Other psychiatric conditions, such as mood disorders and anxiety disorders, also appear at a higher rate in schizophrenia.

BIOLOGICAL TREATMENT

Antipsychotic medication is the first-line treatment for schizophrenia and is most effective when used in conjunction with psychological and social interventions. For youth with schizophrenia, there is generally no convincing evidence to suggest that any particular antipsychotic medication, either first generation or second generation (with the exception of clozapine), is more effective or safe than any other antipsychotic medication. The Food and Drug Administration (FDA) has approved risperidone, aripiprazole, quetiapine, paliperidone, and olanzapine for the treatment of schizophrenia in children under the age of 13 years, while haloperidol and molindone have been approved for adolescents over the age of 13 years. Given its high risk of weight gain and other metabolic disturbances, olanzapine should not be used as the first antipsychotic in children and adolescents. An adequate trial of an antipsychotic is defined as six weeks of continuous treatment at a therapeutic dose. If the initial antipsychotic is ineffective, another antipsychotic medication should be initiated. Medication for the treatment of schizophrenia is needed long term, as the risk of relapse is high when medications are discontinued. Long-acting injectable (LAI) antipsychotics should be discussed with patients and families at all phases of the illness, including the critical period of the first two to five years of illness. Since nonadherence to antipsychotic medications is common and associated with poor outcomes, the early introduction of LAI antipsychotics can dramatically improve a child's or adolescent's symptom control and functioning.

For individuals prescribed antipsychotic medications, patients should be monitored for side effects including metabolic changes, extrapyramidal symptoms (EPSs), and sedation. In particular, it is important to obtain a full metabolic profile (body mass index, waist circumference, lipid levels, blood pressure, fasting glucose, and hemoglobin A1c) at baseline before the initiation of a second-generation antipsychotic, with regular follow-up of these parameters. It is imperative to educate patients on a healthy diet, routine exercise, and smoking cessation. Patients receiving antipsychotic medications should be evaluated for EPSs, including tardive dyskinesia, with regular neurologic motor examinations, assessing for changes in tone and the presence of involuntary, spontaneous movements. Other less common side effects include sexual dysfunction, hyperprolactinemia, electrocardiographic changes, and elevated liver function test levels.

As in adult-onset schizophrenia, clozapine has superior efficacy in treatment-resistant schizophrenia in children and adolescents. However, it is considered a second-line medication for schizophrenia and should only be used in the setting of refractory cases, defined as a failure of two or more first-line antipsychotic medications. Its side effect profile, especially its risk of causing agranulocytosis, necessitates careful monitoring of white blood cell (WBC) and absolute neutrophil counts (ANCs). These labs should be measured at baseline before initiating treatment, weekly for the first six months of treatment, biweekly for the next six months, and then monthly thereafter.

PSYCHOLOGICAL TREATMENT

Psychological interventions are important adjuncts to pharmacological intervention. Particularly, cognitive behavioral therapy (CBT) for psychosis can help address maladaptive thought processes, decrease symptoms, and improve adherence to medications. In addition to CBT, psychoeducation, problem-solving seminars, and family interventions have been associated with lower rates of rehospitalization among adolescents with schizophrenia.

Support for caregivers of children and adolescents with schizophrenia can be instrumental in aiding improving their understanding of the disorder and helping families cope with the diagnosis. Psychoeducation can help provide families with information that can promote a home environment that will be less likely to exacerbate symptoms and trigger a relapse. The American Academy of Child and Adolescent Psychiatry (AACAP) has published a Facts for Families article on schizophrenia containing useful information for parents and caregivers (https://www.aacap.org/AACAP/Families_and_Youth/Facts_for_Families/FFF-Guide/Schizophrenia-In-Children-049.aspx). In general, more nurturing and positive environments are associated with better outcomes than those characterized by negativity.

SOCIAL TREATMENT

An integrated approach that addresses education, employment, and social domains can be efficacious in improving treatment adherence, quality of life, and symptom severity. Specifically, some youth can benefit from Individualized Educational Programs (IEPs) or vocational training programs. Socially, interventions such as life skills, problem-solving, and social skills training can help address these deficits.

KEY POINTS TO REMEMBER

- Schizophrenia presenting before the age of 14 years is rare, with most cases presenting between the ages of 14 and 30 years.
- A prodromal phase, characterized by a decline in function, often precedes active symptoms (delusions, hallucinations, disorganized thoughts/behaviors).
- The primary treatment for schizophrenia is antipsychotic medications, with the choice of initial treatment guided by age and side effect profile.
- Adjunctive psychological and social interventions can improve treatment adherence and clinical outcomes.

Further Reading

Kodish I, McClellan JM. Early onset schizophrenia. In: Dulcan, MK, ed., *Dulcan's Textbook of Child and Adolescent Psychiatry*. Arlington, VA: American Psychiatric Association Publishing, 2016:389–408.

Marder SR, Cannon TD. Schizophrenia. *New Engl J Med* 2019;381(18):1753–1761.

McClellan JM, Stock S, American Academy of Child and Adolescent Psychiatry Committee on Quality Issues. Practice parameter for the assessment and treatment of children and adolescents with schizophrenia. *J Am Acad Child Adolesc Psychiatry* 2013;52(9):976–990.

Starling J, Feijo I. Schizophrenia and other psychotic disorders of early onset. In: Rey JM, ed., *IACAPAP e-Textbook of Child and Adolescent Mental Health*. Geneva: International Association for Child and Adolescent Psychiatry and Allied Professions, 2012:Chapter H.5, p. 1–22.

Zaim N, Findling RL, Sun A. Antipsychotics for treatment of adolescent onset schizophrenia: A review. *Curr Treat Options Psychiatry* 2020;7(1):23–28.

7 Several weeks of low mood, decreased appetite, and poor sleep after changing schools

Mila N. Grossman

A 14-year-old girl presents to her pediatrician for an annual wellness visit. While in the waiting room, the patient completed a Patient Health Questionnaire-modified for Adolescents (PHQ-A) form, a depression screening tool modified for adolescents. Her PHQ-A score of 13 is within the range of "moderate depression." Given these findings, the pediatrician spends additional time during the visit exploring recent mood symptoms.

During one-on-one evaluation, the patient reports a three-week history of low mood, decreased appetite, impaired concentration, and poor sleep. She notes she is struggling with her recent transition to a new school. She becomes tearful during the conversation and displays a dysphoric affect. She denies suicidal ideation or a history of self-injurious behavior. A discussion with the patient's mother reveals that she has been irritable and spending more time in her room. She is no longer participating in family outings, which she previously enjoyed, and is arguing more with her sister. She notes that the patient is typically a straight A student; however, she has recently missed several days of school and her grades are suffering.

What Do You Do Now?

The patient is suffering from a major depressive episode characterized by depressed mood and multiple neurovegetative symptoms. Symptoms are impacting the patient's ability to function in multiple domains, notably interfering with her academic performance and relationships with her family members. She is not experiencing suicidal ideation or engaging in self-harm; however, close monitoring and treatment will be important to prevent worsening symptoms of depression and other possible sequelae of untreated depression including substance use, disordered eating, and suicidal behaviors.

EPIDEMIOLOGY

Major depressive disorder (MDD) is one of the most common psychiatric disorders among children and adolescents. Prevalence rates for depressive episodes over a one-year period vary significantly by age: 5% of 12-year-olds, 13% of 14-year-olds, and 17% of 17-year-olds. Prior to puberty, rates of depression are relatively equal between girls and boys, but after puberty, girls are approximately two times more likely to be affected. Despite the relatively high prevalence, it is estimated that less than half of adolescents with depression receive a diagnosis or treatment. Depressive episodes in youth last for an average of six to nine months if left untreated. Major depressive disorder is usually a chronic or relapsing-remitting condition, where about 50% of youth with an initial depressive episode experience a relapse. A substantial proportion of children and adolescents who experience depressive episodes will continue to experience symptoms into adulthood. An earlier age of onset of depression is associated with a more severe and chronic course. Youth presenting with a major depressive episode must be closely monitored for the emergence of symptoms of mania, as between 20% and 40% of children who experience a depressive episode will develop bipolar disorder.

Risk factors for pediatric depression include genetics, chronic medical illness, and environmental stressors. Children and adolescents with a family history of depression or other mental illness, particularly in first-degree relatives, are at increased risk of experiencing MDD. In addition, individuals with psychiatric comorbidities such as anxiety disorders, attention-deficit/hyperactivity disorder (ADHD), and substance use disorders are at higher risk for developing MDD. Medical illnesses such as thyroid disease, viral infections, head injuries, and other chronic illnesses can also precipitate or exacerbate depressive episodes. Psychosocial stressors also contribute to the development of depression. Examples include the loss of a close friend or family member, parental separation or divorce, moving homes or school changes, and bullying or other trauma. Finally, children and adolescents from low socioeconomic backgrounds and minority communities experience higher rates of depression and are less likely to access treatment.

SIGNS AND SYMPTOMS

According to the *Diagnostic and Statistical Manual of Mental Disorders*, Fifth Edition (DSM-5), MDD is characterized by a history of one or more depressive episodes in the absence of a history of mania. A depressive episode is defined by the presence of five or more symptoms with at least one of the symptoms being depressed and/or irritable mood OR anhedonia (loss of pleasure). The presence of predominantly irritable rather than depressed mood is specific to children and adolescents and differs from adult criteria for MDD. Other symptoms include problems with sleep (insomnia or hypersomnia), changes in appetite (significant weight loss or failure to gain weight as expected or significant weight gain), psychomotor retardation or agitation, decreased energy or fatigue, feelings of guilt or worthlessness, impaired concentration, and thoughts about death or suicide. Symptoms must be present for at least two weeks and cause significant distress or impairment in the individual's ability to function. Symptoms cannot be the result of another medical condition or attributable to the effects of medication or substance use.

The DSM-5 uses specifiers to further characterize depressive episodes including anxious distress, atypical features, melancholic features, and psychotic features. Of note, children and adolescents are more likely to experience depressive episodes with atypical features, characterized by mood reactivity (improved mood in the setting of positive stimuli), increased appetite, and hypersomnia.

Children and adolescents with depression may present differently than adults. Pediatric depression is more commonly characterized by irritability or cranky mood rather than by feelings of sadness or low mood. Children may have difficulty identifying or describing their mood as sad. They also often have a difficult time identifying anhedonia. This symptom may be reported by parents who observe that their child has decreased interest in previously enjoyable activities. Youth experiencing anhedonia often report pervasive feelings of boredom. In addition, children are more likely to report physical complaints such as headache or abdominal pain. School performance often suffers, and children and adolescents are more likely to experience school avoidance. Other behavioral correlates include problems with peer and/or family relationships, withdrawal from social activities, sleep problems, and engaging in risky behaviors (e.g., promiscuity or substance use). Children and adolescents with depression have fewer melancholic symptoms such as significant weight loss, excessive guilt, and lack of reactivity to positive events; delusions; and suicide attempts compared to adults with depression.

ASSESSMENT

The United States Preventive Services Task Force recommends universal annual depression screening in patients ages 12 to 18 years. Primary care physicians often employ depression screening tools (such as the PHQ-A) to identify high-risk patients; however, scoring high on a questionnaire does not confirm a diagnosis of MDD. If a child or adolescent is identified as high risk, either by a screening tool or their presenting symptoms, a thorough evaluation is necessary to confirm the diagnosis. Assessment for depression begins with a one-on-one interview to identify whether symptoms of depression are present and their overall impact on the patient's functioning. Collateral information from families, caregivers, and teachers is also critical for establishing a diagnosis in children and adolescents.

In addition to a thorough psychiatric interview and mental status examination, the evaluation should include a medical history, physical examination, and focused laboratory studies including thyroid-stimulating hormone, complete blood count, comprehensive metabolic panel, vitamin B12, folate, and urine toxicology to rule out medical and/or substance-related causes. Clinicians should also screen for comorbid psychiatric conditions such as anxiety, ADHD, substance use disorders, disruptive behavior disorders, and eating disorders.

The evaluation should also consider potential depressive episode precipitants including recent losses, interpersonal problems at home or at school (e.g., parent-child discord, bullying), trauma, and gender dysphoria. Identification of stressors can help guide treatment. Clinicians must also assess for any acute safety concerns including urges to self-harm, recent self-injurious behavior, suicidal ideation, and homicidal ideation. The patient should be asked directly about suicidal ideation, plans, and past attempts. Providers should also seek to understand the patient's specific risk and protective factors for self-harm or suicide. Common factors that increase the risk for suicide include a history of self-injurious behaviors, previous suicide attempts, a family history of completed suicide, substance use, and ongoing untreated symptoms of depression. Protective factors include engagement in mental health treatment, treatment responsivity, robust social supports, and the ability to use adaptive coping skills. The provider should also help identify ways to increase the child's safety, including recommending that parents remove guns from the home and ensure that the child has adequate supervision.

The initial assessment and diagnosis of MDD is often made by the patient's primary care doctor; however, in situations where the diagnosis is not clear or symptoms are severe, the patient should be referred to a pediatric psychiatrist or other mental health specialist for further evaluation and treatment.

LEVEL OF CARE

Treatment of pediatric depression occurs in a variety of settings including outpatient care, partial hospitalization programs, residential programs, and inpatient care. Attempts should be made to provide care in the least restrictive setting possible, while maintaining safety and efficacy. When determining the most appropriate level of care, consideration should be given to safety concerns, the severity of depression (e.g., presence of psychotic symptoms; insight into illness), motivation for treatment, the level of parental support, and the child/family's preferences. Children and adolescents with active suicidal ideation, homicidal ideation, severe psychotic symptoms, or significant impairment in functioning typically require inpatient hospitalization. If there is no imminent risk of suicide but the severity of depression is of concern, then a partial hospitalization program may be appropriate.

BIOLOGICAL TREATMENT

Once a diagnosis of pediatric depression is made, it is important to assess the severity of the illness. In cases of mild to moderate depression, it is often appropriate for providers to recommend a period of active monitoring, support, and psychotherapy interventions before initiating psychopharmacologic interventions. Active monitoring should last for a maximum of two to four weeks with weekly or biweekly visits before implementing treatment interventions with either psychotherapy or medications. Mild to moderate cases of depression may respond to psychotherapy alone. The use of antidepressant medications can accelerate the rate of treatment response and they are often needed in moderate or severe cases of depression.

There are currently two Food and Drug Administration (FDA)-approved medications for the treatment of pediatric depression: fluoxetine in children and adolescents ages eight years and older and escitalopram in adolescents ages 12 years and older. Both of these medications are selective serotonin reuptake inhibitors (SSRIs), which increase the level of the neurotransmitter serotonin in the brain. Selective serotonin reuptake inhibitors typically take four to six weeks to take full effect; ultimately, 55% to 65% of pediatric patients taking an SSRI will experience relief of depressive symptoms. The American Academy of Child and Adolescent Psychiatry (AACAP) recommends that the medication be continued for one year after full remission of symptoms with monthly monitoring.

Common side effects of SSRIs include gastrointestinal symptoms (nausea, stomachaches, and/or diarrhea), headaches, agitation, sleep disturbance, irritability, and behavioral activation. These side effects are typically mild and self-resolve over time. Notably, in 2004, the FDA issued a black-box warning indicating that antidepressant medications were associated with an increased risk of suicidal thinking and behavior in children and adolescents. In a review of over 2,000 youth, antidepressant medications were associated with increased rates of suicidal thinking/behavior compared with placebo (4% vs. 2%). There were no completed suicides in any of the studies. While the initiation of an SSRI may slightly increase the risk for suicidal thoughts and behaviors, the benefits of treating the underlying depression almost certainly outweigh these risks, as untreated depression also increases the risk for suicide. That being said, close monitoring for the emergence of increased suicidality is imperative when starting an SSRI. Finally, children and adolescents who are being treated with antidepressants should be closely monitored for the emergence of symptoms of mania (e.g., elevated, expansive, or irritable mood; decreased need for sleep; increased energy; and increased activity).

Although there are only two FDA-approved medications for the treatment of pediatric depression, the use of other antidepressants is a common and accepted clinical practice. While the two FDA-approved SSRIs are typically first-line medications for pediatric depression, other SSRIs (e.g., citalopram, sertraline) or non-SSRI classes of antidepressant medications (e.g., serotonin norepinephrine reuptake inhibitors, bupropion, or mirtazapine) may be used if first-line medication options are ineffective or intolerable. If necessary, the combination of two antidepressants or augmenting an antidepressant with a second-generation antipsychotic may be used. Tricyclic antidepressants (TCAs) and monoamine oxidase inhibitors (MAOIs) are not recommended as first- or second-line treatment options because they have not been proven to be effective in youth and are associated with more serious side effects.

The AACAP has published a medication guide for depression that can be distributed to parents (https://www.aacap.org/App_Themes/AACAP/docs/resource_centers/resources/med_guides/DepressionGuide-web.pdf).

PSYCHOSOCIAL TREATMENT

Pediatric depression can be distressing for patients and their family members. An important part of treatment is providing psychoeducation about the symptoms of depression, the typical clinical course, and treatment options. The AACAP's Facts for Families can be used to guide this discussion (https://www.aacap.org/AACAP/Families_and_Youth/Facts_for_Families/FFF-Guide/The-Depressed-Child-004.aspx). Parents, caregivers, and teachers can play a pivotal role in pediatric depression treatment by providing support and helping the child or adolescent to reduce stress. Particular attention should be paid to promoting regular physical exercise, good sleep hygiene, and a healthy diet.

Psychotherapy alone or in combination with antidepressant therapy has been proven to be effective in the treatment of pediatric depression. For mild to moderate cases of depression, a trial of psychotherapy should be considered as a first-line treatment before considering pharmacologic interventions. Mild to moderate depressive episodes may respond to therapy alone. The Treatment for Adolescents with Depression Study (TADS) compared the effectiveness of fluoxetine, cognitive behavioral therapy (CBT), and their combination in adolescents with MDD. The results demonstrated that in adolescents with moderate to severe depression, combined treatment was superior to either monotherapy. The most well-studied and efficacious therapies for pediatric depression are CBT and interpersonal psychotherapy (IPT). Cognitive behavioral therapy targets a patient's thoughts and behaviors to improve their mood. Interpersonal psychotherapy works by focusing on improving interpersonal relationships with friends and family and developing interpersonally effective problem-solving skills. Other types of therapy such as dialectical behavioral therapy, supportive therapy, and family therapy may also be helpful.

KEY POINTS TO REMEMBER

- Pediatric depression occurs in approximately 13% of adolescents in the United States.
- While the prevalence of pediatric depression is high, less than 50% of affected patients receive adequate treatment.
- Irritable mood is often a hallmark of pediatric depression; other symptoms include anhedonia, changes in sleep, decreased appetite, impaired concentration, boredom, and social isolation.
- Suicide is the second leading cause of death among children ages 10 to 14 years and 15 to 19 years.
- Treatment for pediatric depression includes both psychotherapy and antidepressant interventions.

Further Reading

Cheung AH, Zuckerbrot RA, Jensen PS, et al. Guidelines for adolescent depression in primary care (GLADPC): Part II. Treatment and ongoing management. *Pediatrics* 2018;141(3):e20174082.

Delph SS, McDonagh MS. Depression in children and adolescents: Evaluation and treatment. *Am Fam Physician* 2019;100(10):609–617.

Mojtabai R, Olfson M, Han B. National trends in the prevalence and treatment of depression in adolescents and young adults. *Pediatrics* 2016;138(6):e20161878.

O'Connor BC, Lewandowski RE, Rodriguez S, et al. Usual care for adolescent depression from symptom identification through treatment initiation. *JAMA Pediatr* 2016;170:373.

Zuckerbrot RA, Cheung A, Jensen PS, et al. Guidelines for adolescent depression in primary care (GLAD-PC): Part I. Practice preparation, identification, assessment, and initial management. *Pediatrics* 2018;141(3):e20174081.

8 An episode of giddy, irritable mood with increased energy and goal-directed activity

Joshua R. Smith

A 17-year-old boy presents to the psychiatry clinic due to a dramatic change in mood and behavior over the past two weeks. He describes his mood as "better than ever." His parents note that while he has seemed giddy, he has also been quick to anger. He's had little sleep yet has excessive amounts of energy during the day. He has been speaking so rapidly that it is difficult to follow his train of thought. He denies using any substances.

In middle school, he was depressed and treated with fluoxetine. His depressive symptoms resolved after two months and the medication was discontinued after one year. At baseline, his parents describe him as a pleasant and "easygoing" teenager.

On psychiatric assessment, he cannot stay still. It is difficult to interrupt him as he talks about numerous projects he wants to begin. He cannot understand why his parents are concerned and states that he feels "better than ever," despite appearing quite irritable.

What Do You Do Now?

The patient is likely suffering from a manic episode, meeting criteria for bipolar disorder. Rapid identification, diagnosis, and treatment are paramount, as untreated symptoms can have dire consequences including legal problems, inability to participate in academic activities, and psychiatric hospitalization.

EPIDEMIOLOGY

The reported prevalence of pediatric bipolar disorder has ranged from 0.6% to 2.9%, with one meta-analysis of international studies reporting a prevalence rate of 1.8%. The most well-established risk factor for bipolar disorder in children and adolescents is a family history of bipolar disorder. Common premorbid symptoms that exist prior to developing bipolar disorder include irritability, depression, anxiety, hyperactivity, and inattention. Comorbid psychiatric conditions are common and include substance use disorders, anxiety disorders, oppositional defiant disorder, conduct disorder, antisocial personality disorder, and attention-deficit/hyperactivity disorder (ADHD).

SIGNS AND SYMPTOMS

According to the *Diagnostic and Statistical Manual of Mental Disorders*, Fifth Edition (DSM-5), the diagnostic criteria for mania include a distinct period of abnormally and persistently elevated, expansive, or irritable mood and persistently increased activity or energy that are present most of the day, nearly every day, lasting at least one week. At least three of the following accompanying symptoms (four if mood is only irritable) must be present: inflated self-esteem or grandiosity, decreased need for sleep, more talkative than usual or pressure to keep talking, flight of ideas, distractibility, increase in goal-directed activity or psychomotor agitation, and excessive involvement in activities that have a high potential for painful consequences. Additionally, the symptoms must be severe and cause marked impairments in functioning, necessitate hospitalization, or be accompanied by psychotic features. To meet criteria for a hypomanic episode, the patient must exhibit the same symptoms for at least four consecutive days, but they must not be so severe that there is marked impairment in functioning or the need for hospitalization.

The accurate distinction between mania and hypomania is important when diagnosing specific subtypes of bipolar disorder. Bipolar I disorder is diagnosed when the patient meets criteria for a manic episode. The manic episode may have been preceded by and may be followed by hypomanic or major depressive episodes. A diagnosis of bipolar II disorder requires the patient to have met criteria for at least one past or current hypomanic episode and one past or current major depressive episode.

Clinical presentations of pediatric bipolar disorder are often heterogenous and can differ from adult presentations. In children, the mood state can alternate between euphoric mania and melancholic depression. However, severe aggression is common (e.g., kicking, hitting, biting, spitting) regardless of the mood state and, when present, is highly impairing. Furthermore, children with bipolar disorder are seldom euthymic, alternating between episodes of mania and depression. Mood episodes with mixed features (three nonoverlapping symptoms of opposite polarity) are more common in children and adolescents with bipolar disorder, occurring in greater than 80% of affected youth. Psychotic symptoms are more common in children and adolescents, while decreased need for sleep is less common than in adults. Grandiosity in children typically presents as an extreme disregard for rules and overconfidence, characterized by taking on age-inappropriate tasks or defying authority figures. Mood episodes in pediatric bipolar disorder are marked by irritability, rapid mood fluctuations, and mixed symptoms of depression and mania. Distinct manic and major depressive episodes classically seen in adult-onset bipolar disorder are less common.

ASSESSMENT

The diagnosis of bipolar disorder is made by completing a detailed history of presenting symptoms obtained from the patient and caregivers in conjunction with conducting a mental status examination. Pertinent findings on the mental status examination include irritability, impulsivity, increased verbal output, and psychomotor agitation. These findings are sensitive but not specific for mania, given their presence in myriad other conditions including ADHD, disruptive behavior disorders, neurodevelopmental disorders, and posttraumatic stress disorder. Additional mental status examination findings including sexualized behaviors or thought disorganization are suggestive of pediatric bipolar disorder but may also occur in other conditions. Key clinical features that distinguish mania from other psychiatric disorders include episodicity, a clear departure from baseline functioning, and severity. To qualify for a diagnosis of mania, the mood and associated symptoms described in the DSM-5 must be present most of the time for at least several days in a row. Additionally, the symptoms must be severe enough that they represent a clear change from baseline mood and functioning that is readily observable by the child's caregivers. The degree of irritability in pediatric mania is very severe, often including physical aggression that would otherwise be uncharacteristic of the child.

Regarding the differential diagnoses, along with characterization of various bipolar disorder subtypes as discussed earlier, other psychiatric disorders should be ruled out. If psychotic symptoms are present, a primary psychotic disorder such as schizophrenia should be included in the differential diagnosis. However, primary psychotic disorders are less common in children and are typically preceded by a prodromal period of declining social and academic functioning, which is not characteristic of bipolar disorder. The diagnoses of ADHD and anxiety disorders should also be considered, although these are less likely to be characterized by psychosis, chronic irritability, and rapidly changing mood states. Finally, disruptive mood dysregulation disorder shares features of mania, such as severe temper outbursts and angry/irritable mood, but cannot be codiagnosed if the child meets full criteria for mania or hypomania.

An important component of the medical workup of bipolar disorder is a urine toxicology screen to rule out substance-induced mood symptoms. However, many adolescents experience an increase in substance use during or secondary to mania, highlighting the importance of inquiring about the timeframe and quantity of substance use.

LEVEL OF CARE

The initial evaluation of a child or adolescent with suspected bipolar disorder should include a safety assessment as well as an evaluation of the severity of the condition to determine the most appropriate level of care. If the patient's symptoms of suicidal ideation, impulsivity, irritability, or risky behaviors place themselves or others at an elevated imminent risk for harm, the patient should be treated in an inpatient setting. Partial hospital programs may be appropriate in cases where there is severe symptomatology and the child is unable to function in the school setting but safety can be adequately maintained in the community.

BIOLOGICAL TREATMENT

Pharmacological management of bipolar disorder in children and adolescents is the cornerstone of treating acute mood episodes and preventing future episodes. The Food and Drug Administration (FDA)-approved treatments of manic or mixed episodes in patients 10 to 17 years old include the following second-generation antipsychotics: risperidone, aripiprazole, quetiapine, olanzapine, and asenapine. Lithium is also FDA approved for the treatment of manic or mixed episodes in adolescents. The use of second-generation antipsychotics is associated with greater improvement in symptoms of mania compared with traditional mood stabilizers (e.g., valproic acid, lithium, carbamazepine). The FDA-approved treatments for major depressive episodes in pediatric bipolar disorder include the second-generation antipsychotic lurasidone and the combination of olanzapine and fluoxetine. Medications with a strong evidence base for the treatment of major depressive episodes in adult-onset bipolar disorder additionally include lithium, lamotrigine, and quetiapine.

Despite active treatment, relapse rates are high, at approximately 60% in the 18 months following a mood episode, even when the patient is receiving treatment with a mood stabilizer. Thus, the vast majority of patients require long-term treatment with mood stabilizers to minimize the risk of future episodes of depression and/or mania, increasing their cumulative exposure to medications and risk for side effects. For second-generation antipsychotics, metabolic syndrome is a common complication. A baseline waist circumference, body mass index, blood pressure, hemoglobin A1c, and lipid panel should be obtained prior to initiating a second-generation antipsychotic and monitored regularly. A series of parallel trials that compared weight gain over a period of eight weeks in open-label second-generation antipsychotic monotherapy in children (ages five to 14 years) with bipolar disorder demonstrated that olanzapine was associated with the most weight gain (>5 kg), while ziprasidone was associated with the least weight gain (1 kg). The weight gain associated with risperidone, quetiapine, and aripiprazole was similar and intermediate. Extrapyramidal symptoms including tardive dyskinesia are another possible complication of long-term treatment with antipsychotics, and children should be regularly assessed for these adverse effects. For lithium, baseline laboratory tests should be obtained including a complete blood count, thyroid function tests, urinalysis, basic metabolic panel including renal function tests, serum calcium levels, and pregnancy test in females of childbearing age. Once a stable lithium dose is obtained, continued periodic laboratory monitoring should be conducted with particular focus on thyroid-stimulating hormone and creatinine.

As previously discussed, psychiatric comorbidity is common and should also be treated. After mood stabilization is achieved, stimulants may be cautiously considered for ADHD, as well as medications for refractory anxiety or depression.

PSYCHOSOCIAL TREATMENT

Patient and family psychoeducation regarding the etiology, symptoms, medications, and prognosis of bipolar disorder in children and adolescents is an important starting point for treatment. The American Academy of Child and Adolescent Psychiatry (AACAP) has published a Facts for Families article, which can be distributed to parents (https://www.aacap.org/AACAP/Families_and_Youth/Facts_for_Families/FFF-Guide/Bipolar-Disorder-In-Children-And-Teens-038.aspx). Individual psychotherapy for children and adolescents targeted at increasing emotion regulation, problem-solving skills, and communication skills is the most well-established treatment associated with reduced symptomatology. These therapeutic skills can be taught and reinforced through interpersonal therapy (IPT), cognitive behavioral therapy (CBT), or dialectical behavioral therapy (DBT). Social rhythm therapies that support the implementation of regular, daily patterns of activity to improve and stabilize mood have been demonstrated to be effective for adults with bipolar disorder. A pilot trial integrating principles of IPT with social rhythm therapy adapted for adolescents with bipolar disorder demonstrated feasibility, acceptability, and improvement in psychiatric symptoms. Additionally, since rates of comorbid anxiety disorders are high in children and adolescents with bipolar disorder, and commonly used first-line antianxiety medications such as selective serotonin reuptake inhibitors and serotonin norepinephrine reuptake inhibitors may worsen mood stability, a trial of evidence-based psychotherapy (e.g., CBT) should be considered for treating comorbid anxiety disorder prior to initiating pharmacotherapy.

KEY POINTS TO REMEMBER

- Pediatric bipolar disorder most often presents with a rapidly fluctuating mixed mood state characterized by irritability, impulsivity, rapid speech, and psychomotor agitation.
- Compared to adult-onset bipolar disorder, psychotic symptoms are more common in youth, while decreased need for sleep is less common.
- Pharmacological management with second-generation antipsychotics is considered first-line treatment for mania.
- Relapse rates are high, even among patients receiving treatment.
- Family psychoeducation, skill building, and community engagement may decrease overall symptom burden.

Further Reading

Goldstein BI, Birmaher B, Carlson GA, et al. The International Society for Bipolar Disorders Task Force Report on pediatric bipolar disorder: Knowledge to date and directions for future research. *Bipolar Disord* 2017;19(7):524–543.

Liu HY, Potter MP, Woodworth KY, et al. Pharmacologic treatments for pediatric bipolar disorder: A review and meta-analysis. *J Am Acad Child Adolesc Psychiatry* 2011;50(8):749–762.e39.

McClellan J, Kowatch R, Findling RL. Practice parameter for the assessment and treatment of children and adolescents with bipolar disorder. *J Am Acad Child Adolesc Psychiatry* 2007;46(1):107–125.

Serra G, Uchida M, Battaglia C, et al. Pediatric mania: The controversy between euphoria and irritability. *Curr Neuropharmacol* 2017;15(3):386–393.

Van Meter AR, Burke C, Kowatch RA, et al. Ten-year updated meta-analysis of the clinical characteristics of pediatric mania and hypomania. *Bipolar Disord* 2016;18(1):19–32.

Vaudreuil CAH, Faraone SV, Di Salvo M, et al. The morbidity of subthreshold pediatric bipolar disorder: A systematic literature review and meta-analysis. *Bipolar Disord* 2019;21(1):16–27.

Yapici Eser H, Taşkıran AS, Ertınmaz B, et al. Anxiety disorders comorbidity in pediatric bipolar disorder: A meta-analysis and meta-regression study. *Acta Psychiatr Scand* 2020;141(4):327–339.

9 Chronically irritable mood with frequent temper outbursts

Lauren N. Deaver

A nine-year-old boy presents for an initial psychiatric evaluation of chronically irritable mood and disruptive behavior at home and at school. Over the past year, he has had severe temper tantrums that occur most days of the week, lasting between five and 10 minutes. During these tantrums, he screams, cries, and often pushes others. At school, he throws objects and tries to run out of the classroom when he is upset. Between episodes, he remains irritable and is often described as "cranky" by other people. He has been suspended from school three times since the school year started due to physical fights with other students.

The patient shrugs when asked to talk about the temper tantrums and his mood. When the subject is shifted to other topics such as the family dog, he brightens a bit and talks in full, fluent sentences. His mother reports he has always been hyperactive and distractible. His developmental history and medical history are unremarkable.

What Do You Do Now?

The patient is suffering from disruptive mood dysregulation disorder (DMDD), categorized as a depressive disorder in the *Diagnostic and Statistical Manual of Mental Disorders*, Fifth Edition (DSM-5). It is characterized by chronic, nonepisodic, irritable mood with frequent and severe temper outbursts across multiple settings. Children and adolescents with DMDD have significant psychosocial impairment, particularly in interpersonal functioning with their parents and siblings. In educational settings, they are frequently suspended from school due to inappropriate behaviors that manifest during temper tantrums. They are at increased risk for learning disabilities, self-injurious behavior, and suicidal ideation. In adulthood, patients with DMDD have a higher risk of major depressive disorder (MDD), anxiety disorders, engaging in risky or illegal behaviors, and job loss.

EPIDEMIOLOGY

Disruptive mood dysregulation disorder is a new diagnostic addition to the DSM-5. In the mid-1990s, a rapid increase in the prevalence of pediatric bipolar disorder occurred when a broader pediatric phenotype of mania was introduced. Because of this, the National Institutes of Health spearheaded efforts to better characterize children and adolescents with chronic and impairing irritability, provisionally naming the syndrome severe mood dysregulation (SMD). Severe mood dysregulation was differentiated from bipolar disorder by its characteristic symptoms of chronic, nonepisodic irritability; exaggerated emotional reactivity; and hyperarousal. Ultimately, analysis of longitudinal data found associations between SMD and developing MDD and generalized anxiety disorder (GAD) in adulthood. Nonepisodic (chronic) irritability in youth has not been found to predict future episodes of mania or a diagnosis of bipolar disorder in adulthood. The core features of DMDD were derived from SMD and are very similar; however, the hyperarousal criteria (e.g., insomnia, distractibility, agitation) of SMD were not included in DMDD.

Prevalence estimates of DMDD range from 0.8% to 5% of children and adolescents. Rates of DMDD are higher in school-aged children compared to preschool-aged children and in males. Half of children with severe, chronic irritability will continue to meet criteria for DMDD one year after the initial diagnosis. The disorder becomes less common as children transition into late adolescence and adulthood.

Risk factors associated with DMDD include maternal postpartum depression, paternal depression, parental history of substance use, recent family divorce, relocation, grief, early childhood trauma, one or both parents not living in the home, and lower parental education level.

SIGNS AND SYMPTOMS

The core feature of DMDD is chronic, severe, and persistent irritability. The two essential components are (1) frequent temper outbursts and (2) persistence across time and setting.

Patients must have recurrent temper outbursts that occur on average three or more times per week. Temper outbursts may be verbal or behavioral including physical aggression toward other people or destroying property. The outbursts are grossly out of proportion in intensity or duration to the provoking situation. The outbursts must also be inconsistent with the patient's developmental level.

Between outbursts, patients remain persistently irritable or angry for most the day, nearly every day. Irritability persists across multiple settings, in at least two of home, school, and with peers. The irritability is also easily observable by others.

Patients must experience symptoms for at least one year without a symptom-free period for longer than three months. The onset of irritability and temper outbursts must occur before the age of 10 years. However, DMDD cannot be diagnosed in children younger than six years or in young adults older than 18 years. The presence of symptoms of mania or hypomania lasting more than one day is an exclusionary criterion.

ASSESSMENT

A thorough clinical evaluation is required for the diagnosis of DMDD. Evaluation of temper outbursts should determine the duration and frequency as well as common behaviors during episodes. Triggers for the outbursts and what helps resolve them should be identified. The predominant mood between outbursts should be assessed for quality, variability, and severity. Since the outbursts and persistently irritable mood must occur across settings, information should be obtained from other informants such as teachers or coaches, in addition to parents.

There are no validated rating scales for the assessment of DMDD. Rating scales used to assess irritability may be helpful but cannot be used in lieu of a detailed description of the outbursts and inter-episode mood quality. Examples of rating scales for irritability include the Affective Reactivity Index (ARI) and the Multidimensional Assessment of Preschool Disruptive Behaviors (MAP-DB), which has also been adapted for use in older children.

It is important to recognize that irritability occurs in multiple other psychiatric conditions that affect children. The differential diagnosis includes bipolar disorder, oppositional defiant disorder (ODD), intermittent explosive disorder (IED), ADHD, MDD, and GAD. Chronically irritable mood and severe outbursts differentiate DMDD from other psychiatric disorders. In bipolar disorder, irritability is episodic, and mood fluctuates. Also, the presence of manic or hypomanic symptoms for greater than one day is an important exclusionary criterion for DMDD. In addition, while many children with DMDD meet criteria for ODD, mood symptoms are a core feature of DMDD but are not required to establish a diagnosis of ODD. If the criteria for both are met, only DMDD should be diagnosed. In IED, temper outbursts are less frequent (minimally two per week in IED vs. three per week in DMDD) and irritability is not present between episodes. Neither irritability nor outbursts are core diagnostic symptoms in ADHD. Although irritability is also a common symptom of MDD in children, severe temper outbursts are more specific to DMDD. Finally, in GAD, irritability or outbursts occur in response to certain anxiety-provoking contexts or phobic triggers. While there are features of DMDD that help distinguish this diagnosis from other psychiatric disorders as summarized previously, it should be noted that DMDD is associated with psychiatric comorbidity, and the patient may concurrently meet diagnostic criteria for more than one psychiatric disorder.

BIOLOGICAL TREATMENT

Since DMDD is a new diagnosis, there are no published randomized controlled medication trials to guide prescribing practices. Similarly, there are no Food and Drug Administration (FDA)-approved treatments for DMDD. Pharmacologic treatment should target core symptoms of DMDD including chronic irritability and behavioral outbursts. The use of selective serotonin reuptake inhibitors (SSRIs) and serotonin norepinephrine reuptake inhibitors (SNRIs) may be considered, given their relatively safe side effect profile, their established efficacy for treating irritability due to pediatric MDD and anxiety disorders, and the growing longitudinal evidence base to suggest a close relationship between DMDD, MDD, and anxiety disorders. Side effects of SSRIs and SNRIs include sedation, insomnia, gastrointestinal symptoms, and behavioral activation. Patients and families should be counseled on the FDA black-box warning regarding increased risk of suicidality associated with antidepressant medications in youth as well as the risk of a "manic" switch. The risk of "unmasking" mania when SSRIs or SNRIs are used to treat DMDD is not thought to be higher than when SSRIs or SNRIs are used to treat MDD or GAD.

The second-generation antipsychotic medications risperidone and aripiprazole are both FDA approved for the treatment of irritability associated with autism spectrum disorder in children and adolescents. They are frequently used clinically off-label to target symptoms of irritability in other psychiatric disorders, with some open-label evidence for efficacy in DMDD. Side effects include weight gain, adverse metabolic effects, and sedation. Long-term use may also cause tardive dyskinesia. Risperidone may also cause hyperprolactinemia.

In patients with comorbid ADHD, optimization of stimulant medications, including methylphenidate and amphetamine compounds, can significantly improve DMDD symptoms. Common side effects include appetite suppression, insomnia, headache, and anxiety. When symptoms of irritability persist after psychostimulants are optimized, the addition of either an SSRI/SNRI or second-generation antipsychotic may be considered.

PSYCHOSOCIAL TREATMENT

Disruptive mood dysregulation disorder is associated with high levels of impairment. Parents should receive psychoeducation regarding the symptoms, course, and management of DMDD. The American Academy of Child and Adolescent Psychiatry (AACAP) has published a Facts for Families article on DMDD, which can be distributed to parents (https://www.aacap.org/AACAP/Families_and_Youth/Facts_for_Families/FFF-Guide/Disruptive-Mood-Dysregulation-Disorder-_DMDD_-110.aspx).

In the face of the very limited empirical evidence base for pharmacologic treatments of DMDD, rigorous implementation of psychosocial interventions is important. Parent training interventions are a critical component of a comprehensive treatment plan. In general, studies assessing children with oppositional behavior have demonstrated that parent training interventions are more effective for younger children than for adolescents, highlighting the importance of early diagnosis and intervention in DMDD. Although parent training should also be offered to parents of adolescents, adding individual psychotherapies may be more beneficial for this age group. Although no head-to-head trials of different types of parent training interventions have been conducted in DMDD, consideration should be given to the use of parent management training (PMT) and collaborative problem solving (CPS) for elementary school-aged and high school-aged children, respectively. In PMT, parents typically attend sessions without their child present. Each session they are taught a new skill to manage challenging behaviors and are offered the opportunity to practice them through role-play with the therapist. Families typically attend approximately 10 weekly sessions. In CPS, a combination of parent-only and parent-child sessions are conducted. The goal of CPS is to help parents and children learn to identify recurrent problems and solve them collaboratively by discussing and implementing mutually acceptable solutions.

Individual therapies may include dialectical behavioral therapy (DBT), interpersonal psychotherapy, or cognitive behavioral therapy. Dialectical behavioral therapy is the psychotherapy with the strongest evidence base for DMDD. Goals of DBT in this context include helping the child or adolescent to develop skills to cope with intense emotions through mindfulness, emotion regulation, and distress tolerance. Interpersonal effectiveness skills are also taught. The patient learns DBT skills in a group setting and also participates in individual therapy sessions. Telephone coaching to reinforce skill use between sessions is also usually available. Importantly, parents are taught these skills in conjunction with their child so that they can also help reinforce skill use outside of therapy. A randomized clinical trial comparing DBT to treatment as usual in children with DMDD demonstrated that

DBT was associated with sustained improvements in behavioral outbursts and angry/irritable mood.

KEY POINTS TO REMEMBER

- Chronic (nonepisodic) irritability in children is associated with the future development of MDD and GAD but not with future episodes of mania or bipolar disorder.
- Hallmark symptoms of DMDD include severe, persistent irritability with frequent temper outbursts in multiple settings with significant functional impairment.
- The psychopharmacologic treatment of DMDD may include SSRIs/SNRIs or second-generation antipsychotics and the treatment target is irritability.
- If ADHD is present, initial treatment should include optimization of stimulant medications.
- Psychotherapeutic interventions including parent training interventions are a critical component of a comprehensive treatment plan.

Further Reading

Brotman MA, Schmajuk M, Rich BA, et al. Prevalence, clinical correlates, and longitudinal course of severe mood dysregulation in children. *Biol Psychiatry* 2006;60(9):991–997.

Copeland W, Angold A, Costello E, et al. Prevalence, comorbidity, and correlates of DSM-5 proposed disruptive mood dysregulation disorder. *Am J Psychiatry* 2013;170(2):173–179.

Kreiger FV, Pheula GF, Coelho R, et al. An open-label trial of risperidone in children and adolescents with severe mood dysregulation. *J Child Adolesc Psychopharmacol* 2011; 21(3):237–243.

Leibenluft E. Severe mood dysregulation, irritability, and the diagnostic boundaries of bipolar disorder in youth. *Am J Psychiatry* 2011;168(2):129–142.

Pan P, Fu A, Yeh C. Aripiprazole/methylphenidate combination in children and adolescents with disruptive mood dysregulation disorder and attention-deficit/ hyperactivity disorder: An open label study. *J Child Adolesc Psychopharmacol* 2018;28(10):682–689.

Perepletchikova F, Nathanson D, Axelrod S, et al. Randomized clinical trial of dialectical behavioral therapy for preadolescent children with disruptive mood dysregulation disorder: Feasibility and outcomes. *J Am Acad Child Adolesc Psychiatry* 2017;56(10):832–840.

Stringaris A, Cohen P, Pine DS, et al. Adult outcomes of youth irritability: A 20-year prospective community-based study. *Am J Psychiatry* 2009;166(9):1048–1054.

Waxmonsky J, Waschbusch D, Belin P, et al. A randomized clinical trial of an integrative group therapy for children with severe mood dysregulation. *J Am Acad Child Adolesc Psychiatry* 2016;55(3):196–207.

10 Limited speech outside the home in a young girl who speaks normally at home

Sumita Sharma

Sarah is a five-year-old girl referred for the assessment of limited speech at school. Sarah's teachers noted she has not been speaking to her instructors or peers since starting kindergarten three months ago. Her parents described her as shy and quiet when outside the home and with strangers. At home she is a "chatterbox" with no difficulty speaking with family members. She has close relationships with her siblings and cousins. Sarah's developmental and medical history were unremarkable. Her parents thought she would "grow out of" her shyness and difficulty speaking at school, but now they are becoming more concerned.

On psychiatric evaluation, Sarah appeared shy with limited eye contact. Her receptive language seemed intact and she answered close-ended questions by nodding or shaking her head. When encouraged to speak, she would either look to her parents or whisper inaudibly. When the psychiatrist offered Sarah a puppet, she was initially inhibited but eventually played interactively, giggling and gesturing.

What Do You Do Now?

This patient was diagnosed with selective mutism (SM), an anxiety disorder of childhood characterized by failure to speak in at least one specific social setting such as school, despite the ability to speak in other, more familiar settings. While patients with SM are able to comprehend and appropriately use speech, they have the persistent inability to speak in certain social situations. Evaluation and treatment of this diagnosis can play a critical role in a child's future academic and social performance by decreasing anxiety, increasing communication, enhancing social interactions, and identifying other comorbid medical or psychiatric issues.

EPIDEMIOLOGY

The prevalence of SM is estimated to be between 0.47% and 0.76% in the United States. The historical literature indicates that SM affects more females than males, but recent studies show a more equal distribution between genders. Symptoms typically begin between three and four years of age and rarely begin after 10 years of age. There is often a delay between onset of symptoms and seeking treatment because they are rarely impairing until the child begins school. Vulnerability factors include inhibited temperament, neurodevelopmental delays, immigration, bilingualism, increased parental control, genetic factors, and environmental triggers (e.g., starting school, trauma). Most children with SM experience substantial symptom improvement with age and the mean duration of illness is eight years. However, a childhood history of SM is associated with residual social and communication deficits in adulthood with lower self-ratings of independence, motivation, and confidence. Adults with a history of childhood SM are also at greater risk of developing anxiety disorders, and it has been postulated that SM may be an early manifestation of social anxiety disorder.

SIGNS AND SYMPTOMS

In the *Diagnostic and Statistical Manual of Mental Disorders*, Fifth Edition (DSM-5), SM is categorized as an anxiety disorder. The diagnostic criteria include consistent failure to speak in specific social contexts that require communication, such as school, despite speaking in other situations. It interferes with daily functioning in educational or occupational achievement and/or social communication. The symptoms must be present for at least one month (not including the first month of school). The inability to speak must not be attributable to the lack of knowledge of, or comfort with, the spoken language required in the social situation and is not better explained by a communication disorder (e.g., stuttering). It may not occur exclusively during the course of autism spectrum disorder (ASD) or a psychotic disorder.

While each individual presents differently, associated symptoms often include excessive shyness, difficulty responding to or initiating speech, freezing or awkward body movements when anxious, poor eye contact, social isolation or withdrawal, fear of embarrassment, prolonged speech latency, clinging to caregivers, temper tantrums, compulsive traits, and oppositional behaviors. Despite the failure to speak, the child's nonverbal communication ability is typically age appropriate across settings and children with SM often exhibit prosocial nonverbal communicative behaviors such as nodding, smiling, or giggling.

Selective mutism frequently co-occurs with other communication (speech and language) delays or disorders. Difficulties can include impairments in pragmatics, voice, fluency, articulation, grammar, or semantics of speech, highlighting the importance of a comprehensive speech and language evaluation if this diagnosis is suspected. Common comorbid psychiatric conditions are social anxiety disorder, generalized anxiety disorder, obsessive-compulsive disorder, mood disorders, oppositional defiant disorder (ODD), ASD, enuresis, and encopresis.

ASSESSMENT

The assessment of SM requires a comprehensive and multimodal approach involving a diagnostic interview with parents and teachers, review of parent-completed rating scales, direct observation of the child, and consideration of other comorbid or exclusionary disorders. The interview with the child's parents should seek to determine the time course of symptom onset and evolution, developmental history, medical history, family history, social history, psychiatric history (including trauma), and previous treatments. Parent interviews should also assess for the presence of other psychiatric comorbidities and medical conditions that negatively impact speech, such as neurologic defects involving the speech centers of the brain or hearing difficulties. Teachers should also be involved in the assessment, as they can provide information about the child's symptoms and functioning in the school environment, level of academic achievement, and relationships with classmates.

There are several validated questionnaires and rating scales for SM that can be used to inform the diagnostic assessment and measure severity. The Selective Mutism Questionnaire collects parent-reported information about the child's ability to speak in three different environments: home, school, and social situations outside of school. Scores can be used as evidence for a possible diagnosis of SM. The Selective Mutism Questionnaire can aid in determining the severity of SM. The Selective Mutism Stages of Communication Comfort Scale is a clinician-rated tool that can be used to describe the initial severity of SM and track progress. This scale describes four stages of communication, ranging from lack of responding and initiating (stage 0) to verbal communication (stage 3). Accurate determination of the severity of SM is important when developing relevant and achievable therapeutic goals.

Directly observing and meeting with a child offers the clinician an understanding of the child's behavior in various environments and the severity of the mutism. Specifically, it establishes a sense of the child's social interaction capabilities, ability to communicate needs (verbally and nonverbally), temperament, and mental status examination findings. The clinical assessment of the child is also used to determine whether there are features suggestive of a neurodevelopmental syndrome, intellectual disability (ID), or medical factors interfering with speech production. Although the child likely may not speak, particularly during the initial visit, the examiner should be prepared to assess the child's relatedness, cognitive abilities, and affect through the use of play or drawing.

Finally, a medical workup should be completed to rule out other causes of inability to speak. A comprehensive physical examination should be completed, assessing for oral-facial abnormalities and dysmorphic features. This should include a hearing and speech and language evaluation. Formal cognitive testing may be indicated to rule out ID, if there is concern for cognitive impairment on clinical assessment. Nonverbal tests of intelligence such as the Leiter scale or Test of Non-verbal Intelligence (TONI) may be used.

The differential diagnosis for SM includes other communication disorders (including expressive and receptive language disorders), ID, hearing impairment, ODD, ASD, mood and anxiety disorders, or psychotic disorders. The unique clinical features of SM include severe impairments with speaking during certain situations despite normal speech in other situations.

BIOLOGICAL TREATMENT

Pharmacotherapy is a well-established treatment for anxiety disorders in children. Because SM falls under the category of anxiety disorders, there has been a rise in the use of psychopharmacology for the treatment of SM. Selective serotonin reuptake inhibitors (SSRIs) are helpful for treating the anxiety-related component of SM. While there are currently no medications approved for the treatment of SM by the Food and Drug Administration (FDA), fluoxetine and sertraline are the two SSRIs that have been most frequently studied in children with SM. This is likely in part due to their well-tolerated side effect profiles and the established FDA approval for the use of these medications in the child and adolescent population for other anxiety disorders. Nonetheless, SSRIs should always be used at the lowest effective dose and patients should be monitored for the presence of side effects. Psychopharmacology should not be the sole treatment component for SM. Medications are often added if the child is not making progress with behavioral interventions alone or if there is another comorbid anxiety or mood disorder. They are most effective when combined with the behavioral treatments outlined next.

PSYCHOSOCIAL TREATMENT

Behavioral therapy and cognitive behavioral therapy (CBT) are the most effective nonpharmacologic interventions for the treatment of SM. Since SM typically affects young children, parents should also be closely involved in behavioral treatments. The goal of behavioral therapy is to create an individualized treatment plan to minimize anxiety, boost self-esteem, and increase social communication. Behavioral therapy involves creating a step-wise plan for the child to speak more in challenging situations.

Specific elements of behavioral therapy for SM can include contingency management (giving tangible rewards to reinforce speaking), shaping reinforcement (rewarding successive approximations of the desired behavior), stimulus fading (gradually altering the social environment), systematic desensitization (patient practices speaking in progressively more anxiety-provoking situations), and social skills training. Cognitive behavioral therapy involves identifying and reframing recurrent anxious thoughts that inhibit the child from speaking. Behavioral therapy approaches as described previously are also used in CBT for SM. Family therapy can be another treatment option, especially when familial factors such as family conflict contribute to the development or maintenance of the child's mutism. These models are multidisciplinary and require the collaboration of parents, teachers, physicians, and therapists (including speech and language therapists, if necessary).

It is not uncommon for the diagnosis of SM to be distressing for a family. It therefore requires extensive psychoeducation regarding signs and symptoms, etiologies, testing, and treatment options. It is imperative that parents are empowered to be involved in the entire treatment course of their child. The Child Mind Institute offers the Parent Guide: How to Help a Child with SM (https://childmind.org/guide/parents-guide-to-sm/), and the Selective Mutism Association has published a helpful Parent's Roadmap (https://www.selectivemutism.org/selective-mutism-a-parents-roadmap/). It may also be beneficial to encourage parents to seek out support through parent support groups. Parent coaching should involve encouraging the parent to set the clear but nonconfrontational expectation that the child speak in social situations. Parents and siblings should also be advised to avoid speaking for the patient.

Psychoeducation about SM should also be provided to the child's teachers. The child's refusal to speak in school settings can lead to academic underachievement, social isolation, and frustration for teachers. Teachers should be informed that the behavior is likely related to anxiety, rather than willful stubbornness. The child's parents and teachers should be encouraged to collaborate to develop strategies to help the child feel more comfortable, continue to make progress academically, and make friends.

- Selective mutism occurs in 0.47% to 0.76% of children and is a childhood anxiety disorder.
- Selective mutism is characterized by the failure to speak in at least one specific social setting, despite the ability to speak in more familiar settings.
- What distinguishes SM from other disorders is the child's ability to maintain verbal communication in certain, more comfortable settings. Children with SM maintain age-appropriate and prosocial nonverbal communication across all settings.
- The primary treatment for SM is behavioral interventions (behavioral therapy or CBT).
- Medications have been found to be most effective when combined with behavioral treatments and may include the use of SSRIs.

Further Reading

Cohan SL, Chavira DA, Stein MB. Psychosocial interventions for children with selective mutism: A critical evaluation of the literature from 1990–2005. *J Child Psychol Psychiatry* 2006;47(11):1085–1097.

Kotrba A. *Selective Mutism: An Assessment and Intervention Guide for Therapists, Educators, and Parents*. Eau Claire, WI: PESI Publishing & Media, 2015.

Mac D. (2015). *Suffering in Silence: Breaking through Selective Mutism*. Bloomington, IN: Balboa Press.

Viana AG, Beidel DC, Rabian B. Selective mutism: A review and integration of the last 15 years. *Clin Psychol Rev* 2009;29(1):57–67.

Wong P. Selective mutism: A review of etiology, comorbidities, and treatment. *Psychiatry (Edgmont)* 2010;7(3):23–31.

11 A fear of dogs

Kevin M. Hill

Mary is a seven-year-old girl who is referred to your clinic for the evaluation of anxiety. Mary's parents share that she has had "panic attacks" for the past year. Her "panic attacks" manifest as shaking and crying hysterically. These began shortly after a neighborhood dog bit her and they only occur when she encounters dogs. Since this incident, Mary has become extremely fearful of all dogs. She now has panic attacks each time the gentle therapy dogs visit her classroom. At first, she could not tolerate being in the same room as them, fleeing the classroom in fear. Now, she avoids going to school on the days the therapy dogs visit, complaining of a stomachache. Her best friend's family recently got a new puppy, and since then Mary has refused to attend playdates at her friend's house, which she previously loved.

What Do You Do Now?

This patient is likely suffering from a common anxiety disorder known as specific phobia. This patient would be diagnosed with animal phobia. Specific phobias consist of persistent, excessive fear or anxiety in response to a specific object or situation. It is important to differentiate specific phobias from common, nonpathological fears of normal development. Unlike fears of normal development, common transient fears that are nonimpairing, specific phobias can lead to a significant and negative impact on the course of a patient's development and daily life.

EPIDEMIOLOGY

The reported prevalence of specific phobias is about 7% to 9% in children and adolescents; however, this may be an underestimate, as many affected individuals never seek clinical attention. Specific phobias tend to be more prominent in females than in males; however, this may be reflective of the cultural stigma of fear expression in males leading to underestimation of prevalence in this group. Behavioral inhibition is a risk factor for specific phobia. Other factors that may contribute include genetic predisposition and a history of fear learning (e.g., observation of parent or other figure exhibiting excessive fear from a neutral stimulus). Specific phobias may arise after a clear inciting event but can also develop spontaneously. Common comorbid psychiatric disorders include generalized anxiety disorder (GAD), separation anxiety disorder, and attention-deficit/hyperactivity disorder (ADHD). Most specific phobias remit spontaneously over the course of several years.

SIGNS AND SYMPTOMS

The *Diagnostic and Statistical Manual of Mental Disorders*, Fifth Edition (DSM-5), describes specific phobia as a marked fear or anxiety about a specific object or situation (termed as the "phobic stimulus"). The phobic stimulus almost always provokes immediate fear or anxiety and is either actively avoided or endured with intense fear or anxiety. The fear or anxiety is out of proportion to the actual danger posed by the specific object or situation and to the sociocultural context. The symptoms evoked by the phobic object/situation must cause clinically significant distress or impairment in functioning. The fear, anxiety, or avoidance must be persistent, typically lasting at least six months. The DSM-5 includes five specifiers for the phobic stimulus: animal (e.g., spiders, insects, dogs), natural environment (e.g., heights, storms, water), blood-injection-injury (e.g., needles, invasive procedures), situational (e.g., airplanes, elevators), and other (e.g., costumed characters, vomiting). It is common for patients to present with more than one specific phobia. Among patients who meet criteria for specific phobia, the mean number of phobic stimuli is three.

An individual patient's fear or anxiety response to the phobic stimulus can vary, depending on situational factors such as the duration of the exposure, whether others are present, and whether certain threatening elements of the phobic stimulus are present (e.g., turbulence during a flight for a patient with a phobia of flying). The degree of the fear or anxiety can range from anticipatory anxiety (worry about future events pertaining to the phobic stimulus) to symptoms of a panic attack when encountering the phobic stimulus. Patients also experience a range of physiological responses to the phobic stimulus, often depending on the phobic stimulus itself. Animal, natural environment, and situational phobic stimuli usually trigger increased arousal of the sympathetic nervous system (e.g., increased blood pressure, rapid heart rate), while blood-injection-injury stimuli tend to trigger vasovagal responses (e.g., decreased blood pressure, decreased heart rate, fainting).

ASSESSMENT

Parents are often unaware of specific phobias since they may manifest as nonspecific behaviors such as crying, tantrums, freezing, or clinging, without an obvious trigger. Because of this, it is important to ask the child directly if there are objects or situations that are frightening to screen for specific phobias. If the child or parent identifies a phobic stimulus, the next step of the assessment is to determine the impact on functioning and the associated degree of impairment. When assessing for the impact on the child's daily functioning, it is often helpful to ask practical questions such as "Do you often find yourself avoiding going to people's homes for fear they may have a dog?" or "How would your life be different if you weren't afraid of dogs?" During the diagnostic interview, it can also be helpful to ask the child questions to assess for physiologic manifestations of anxiety such as "Can you feel your heart beat fast when you are left in the dark?"

It is important to distinguish between transient, developmentally appropriate fears and specific phobias. Examples of common developmentally appropriate fears include loud noises, the dark, being separated from parents, burglars, monsters, and ghosts. To meet the diagnostic threshold for a specific phobia, the fear must be persistent and severe and cause functional impairments. Developmentally normal fears do not affect daily functioning, are transient (less than six months), and usually respond to reassurance or distraction.

Several tools have been developed to aid in the assessment of a child with a suspected specific phobia. An example of such a structured assessment is the Anxiety Disorders Interview Schedule: Child and Parent Versions (ADIS-CP). The ADIS-CP includes a "Feelings Thermometer" for children (rating from 0 to 8), which can be used to aid children in quantifying how severely the phobia impacts their anxiety and functioning. In addition, there are a number of well-studied child and parent self-report instruments to aid in assessment such as the Screen for Child Anxiety Related Emotional Disorders-Revised (SCARED-R). However, it should be emphasized that rating scales cannot replace a thorough psychiatric history and mental status examination for diagnostic assessment and treatment planning. The differential diagnosis for specific phobia among children and adolescents includes developmentally appropriate fear response, GAD, social anxiety disorder, separation anxiety disorder, panic disorder, and agoraphobia.

BIOLOGICAL TREATMENT

The most supported form of treatment for specific phobia is cognitive behavioral therapy (CBT), as discussed previously. Since CBT for specific phobias is highly effective, medications should not be the first-line treatment. However, medications such as selective serotonin reuptake inhibitors may be considered if there are multiple phobic stimuli that are simultaneously impairing, the child is too anxious to participate in CBT, or there is another comorbid anxiety disorder that is interfering.

PSYCHOLOGICAL TREATMENT

The treatment of choice for specific phobia is CBT. The cognitive component of CBT for specific phobia includes identifying and modifying recurrent, maladaptive thoughts about the phobic stimulus, while the behavioral component primarily utilizes exposure techniques. Common recurrent, maladaptive thoughts a child with specific phobia may have include "It's scary" or "Dogs are dangerous." For young children, it is often most effective to collaborate with the child to identify a "more helpful" thought they can repeat to themselves to replace the recurrent, maladaptive thought, such as "I can be brave." Adolescents have greater capacity to identify cognitive distortions ("thinking traps") and weigh the evidence for and against the likelihood of the feared outcome.

The behavioral component of CBT for specific phobia is primarily exposure therapy using systematic desensitization. In systematic desensitization, the child and therapist create a "fear hierarchy" pertaining to the phobic stimulus, which is a list of feared stimuli ordered from the least to the most fear provoking. The child is exposed to the least feared stimulus initially and then gradually works up the hierarchy to the most feared stimulus. Gradual exposure to the feared stimulus allows for extinction of the learned fear response. During an exposure, the child experiences the symptoms of anxiety, tolerates them, and ultimately learns that the symptoms of anxiety do not represent imminent danger. For example, a patient with a fear of dogs may begin the fear hierarchy with looking at a picture of a dog. After the child masters this fear, they might next watch videos of a dog, followed by looking at live dogs from afar, being in the same room as a dog, watching someone else pet a dog, and so on. The end point of the fear hierarchy might be feeding or petting a dog. Each step of the fear hierarchy should be challenging enough to elicit an anxiety response but tolerable enough that exposure to the stimulus can be sustained until the anxiety response diminishes. Each step of the fear hierarchy should be repeated and practiced regularly (ideally several times per week) until it no longer elicits an anxiety response before moving to the next step. Children and adolescents can utilize the cognitive techniques described previously, such as repeating a mantra (e.g., "I can be brave") or recognizing and replacing catastrophic thoughts, during the exposures. Younger children may benefit from receiving positive reinforcers (e.g., sticker charts, tangible rewards, praise) to incentivize practicing exposures. For adolescents, conquering their fear is usually in and of itself a sufficient treatment motivator.

It is worth highlighting that it is also important for the therapist to recruit the child's parents as "cotherapists," as repeating and practicing exposures between therapy sessions is critical to help hasten and sustain the response. Additionally, parents may benefit from modeling and coaching on strategies to support their child during the exposure. To do this effectively, the parent must be able to manage their own distress of allowing the child to experience a fear response (easier said than done!) during an exposure.

SOCIAL TREATMENT

Comprehensive treatment of specific phobias also requires providing psychoeducation to parents and caregivers. It is important to acknowledge that specific phobias are not an uncommon occurrence in children, and they do not necessarily signify an issue with the child's environment. Even children in the most secure and loving environments can develop specific phobias. It is important to remind parents that while it is appropriate to acknowledge the child's reaction to the feared stimulus, they should avoid reinforcing or exacerbating the child's anxiety response. Specific behaviors by parents that tend to exacerbate anxieties are statements that humiliate the child, using the phobic stimulus as a threat, and overprotecting/enabling the child's avoidance of the phobic stimulus. The American Academy of Pediatrics has a helpful website for parents and caregivers to understand more about childhood fears and anxieties (https://www.healthychildren.org/English/health-issues/conditions/emotional-problems/Pages/Understanding-Childhood-Fears-and-Anxieties.aspx).

KEY POINTS TO REMEMBER

- The hallmark of a specific phobia is persistent fear or anxiety caused by exposure to a specific situation or object that is unreasonable or excessive and causes functional impairment.

- Parents may not be aware of the phobic stimulus and specific phobias should be included in the differential diagnosis of nonspecific crying, tantrums, freezing, or clinging.
- If unrecognized, specific phobias can have a severe impact on a child's development and daily life.
- The categories of specific phobias in the DSM-5 are animal, natural environment, blood-injection-injury, situational, and other phobias.
- Cognitive behavioral therapy that includes exposure therapy and systematic desensitization is the mainstay of treatment for specific phobias.

Further Reading

Essau CA, Conradt J, Petermann F. Frequency, comorbidity, and psychosocial impairment of specific phobia in adolescents. *J Clin Child Psychol* 2000;29(2):221–231.

Ollendick TH, King NJ, Muris P. Fears and phobias in children: Phenomenology, epidemiology, and aetiology. *Child Adolesc Ment Health* 2002;7:98–106.

Ollendick TH, Raishevich N, Davis TE 3rd, et al. Specific phobia in youth: Phenomenology and psychological characteristics. *Behav Ther* 2010;41(1):133–141.

Silverman WK, Moreno J. Specific phobia. *Child Adolesc Psychiatr Clin N Am* 2005;14(4):819–843.

12 Trouble being away from mother

Sumita Sharma

Beth is a seven-year-old girl with no prior psychiatric or medical history who presents to her pediatrician's office due to school refusal and accompanying somatic symptoms. Over the past two months, Beth has missed 15 days of school. In the mornings before school, Beth often cries and clings to her mother, complaining of a stomachache. On weekends, Beth does not exhibit any of these behaviors. An evaluation for abdominal pain and vomiting is unremarkable. Upon initial psychiatric evaluation, Beth appears timid and shy. She refuses to separate from her mother during the visit. During the evaluation, she gradually is able to acknowledge she feels "scared" when away from her mother. She worries her mother might be seriously injured when they are apart. Her mother notes that Beth cannot fall asleep in her own bed, crying until she is permitted to sleep in her parents' bed, and often has nightmares of being kidnapped.

What Do You Do Now?

This patient is likely suffering from separation anxiety disorder (SAD), a condition that manifests as extreme fear or worry when a child is separated from their primary attachment figures (usually parents). While difficulty separating is normal in early childhood, it rises to the level of SAD if the associated distress interferes with engaging in age-appropriate behaviors such as attending school. Early diagnosis and intervention are critical, as symptoms can contribute to severe distress, persist into adolescence and young adulthood, and lead to increased risk of future psychopathology. Separation anxiety disorder can also cause impairments in functioning, including social and educational performance. Children and adolescents with SAD are often unable to engage in age-appropriate activities including attending school, visiting their friends' houses, sleeping in their own bed, or going to overnight camp. Finally, treatment of SAD is important because untreated SAD can also negatively impact treatment outcomes of comorbid psychiatric disorders.

EPIDEMIOLOGY

Although SAD most commonly begins in childhood, it can also persist beyond childhood and in certain cases can also begin in adulthood. Estimated prevalence rates for childhood-onset and adult-onset SAD are approximately 4% and 6%, respectively. Data indicates that roughly one-third of childhood-onset cases persist into adulthood. Separation anxiety disorder affects females and males equally. Risk factors for SAD include genetic predisposition (family history of mood, substance use, or somatic symptom and related disorders), attachment style (insecure attachment), parental factors (overprotectiveness, decreased warmth, single-parent households), and environmental factors (life stressors, low socioeconomic status). The course of SAD is typically recurrent, with symptomatic worsening at the beginning of the school year, following holiday breaks, or when transitioning to a new school. Separation anxiety disorder is frequently comorbid with other anxiety disorders (panic disorder, generalized anxiety disorder [GAD], specific phobias), posttraumatic stress disorder, obsessive-compulsive disorder, mood disorders, attention-deficit/hyperactivity disorder, oppositional defiant disorder (ODD), conduct disorder, and substance use disorders.

SIGNS AND SYMPTOMS

The *Diagnostic and Statistical Manual of Mental Disorders*, Fifth Edition (DSM-5), categorizes SAD as an anxiety disorder. The fundamental feature of SAD is developmentally inappropriate and excessive fear or anxiety concerning separation from major attachment figures. This is demonstrated by at least three of recurrent, excessive distress when anticipating or experiencing separation from home or major attachment figures; excessive worry about losing major attachment figures or about possible harm coming to them; excessive worry about experiencing an untoward event that causes separation from a major attachment figure; reluctance or refusal to leave the home because of fear of separation; excessive fear or reluctance of being alone or without major attachment figures; reluctance or refusal to sleep away from home or without being near a major attachment figure; repeated nightmares involving the theme of separation; or repeated complaints of physical symptoms when separation from major attachment figures occurs or is anticipated. Commonly recurring somatic complaints include headaches, stomachaches, nausea, and vomiting. The DSM-5 requires symptoms to be persistent and last for a minimum of four weeks in children and adolescents. They must cause clinically significant distress or impairment.

Historically, SAD was considered to be limited to childhood. However, the DSM-5 removed the age-of-onset criterion and expanded the diagnosis to include adults, recognizing that SAD can begin at any age and that symptoms may persist throughout the lifespan. The presenting signs and symptoms of SAD can differ between children and adults. Symptoms of SAD during childhood and adolescence more commonly manifest as challenging behaviors such as school refusal, temper tantrums, enuresis, or somatic complaints (e.g., headache, abdominal pain, nausea) than cognitive symptoms of anxiety (worry). School refusal is very common among children with SAD, occurring in about three-fourths of this population. If worry does occur, the content is typically centered around fear of separation from parents/caregivers and concerns about untoward events that may result in separation such as accidents, kidnapping, or death. In comparison, symptoms of SAD in adulthood typically consist of worries about separation from intimate partners or children. They are exacerbated by life transitions such as moving, beginning new relationships, or having children. Behavioral reactions to the excessive worry in adults may include making repeated phone calls, following strict schedules, or talking excessively.

ASSESSMENT

The clinical assessment of SAD involves a diagnostic interview of the child and caregivers, review of self-report measures, and evaluation of the parent-child interaction. The initial evaluation should focus on assessing mood and anxiety symptoms, particularly when parent-child separation is anticipated or is occurring. The cognitive (content of worries), somatic (e.g., stomachaches, headaches), and behavioral (e.g., school refusal, temper tantrums) symptoms of anxiety that are elicited by separation or the antici-pation of separation should be assessed. The clinician should also determine how the symptoms of SAD are impairing the child, as this information can be helpful for assessing the severity of illness and building motivation to engage in treatment. During the initial assessment, the clinician will need to weigh the benefits of attempting to separate the child and parent against the risks of disrupting the treatment alliance. It is important to note that it can be developmentally normal for many young children to have difficulty separating from their caregivers in an unfamiliar environment.

A commonly used interview assessment tool is the Anxiety Disorders Interview Schedule: Child and Parent Versions (ADIS-CP), which is a well-established and evidence-supported guide to diagnosing a variety of anxiety disorders in children. Additionally, self-report questionnaires are widely utilized and offer valuable information to confirm the diagnosis, measure the severity of symptoms, and monitor treatment response. Tools such as the Screen for Child Anxiety Related Emotional Disorders-Revised (SCARED-R) or the Spence Children's Anxiety Scale (SCAS) allow for assessment of other childhood anxiety disorders. The Separation Anxiety Assessment Scale (SAAS), Separation Anxiety Avoidance Inventory (SAAI), and Separation Anxiety Scale for Children (SASC) are scales more spe-cific to SAD. Self-report tools can be used to guide clinical assessment but should not replace a thorough clinical evaluation.

The behavioral assessment of the parent-child relationship is an im-portant element in the diagnosis of SAD. Observation should involve witnessing the interactions of the parent and child together, which can begin with observations attained from the waiting room. If the clinician decides to attempt separating the child and parent during the assessment, the clinician should note how well the child tolerates separation and how the parent responds to their child's distress. Finally, children with somatic complaints warrant a thorough physical examination and medical workup to rule out potential underlying medical conditions, such as migraine headaches or gastrointestinal illness as such gastroesophageal reflux disorder.

Separation anxiety disorder can mimic various other psychiatric disorders. The differential diagnosis includes anxiety disorders (most commonly GAD and also panic disorder with or without agoraphobia), ODD, mood disorders, substance use disorder, or, in adults, dependent personality disorder. It is also important to remember that avoidance behaviors may occur or increase during times of stress, such as an inappropriate academic placement or bullying. The hallmark feature of SAD is the predominant fear of separation from a significant attachment figure.

BIOLOGICAL TREATMENT

Pharmacologic treatments for SAD should not be used in the absence of psychosocial interventions. However, medications can be beneficial for patients who do not respond to behavioral interventions or for patients with severe symptoms, including those who are not attending school. In such cases, pharmacotherapy should be used as an adjunct to behavioral or psychotherapeutic interventions. Currently there are no specific medications that are approved by the Food and Drug Administration (FDA) for SAD. However, selective serotonin reuptake inhibitors (SSRIs) are well-established medications for the treatment of anxiety disorders in children and adolescents. Buspirone, a serotonin receptor partial agonist, may also be considered. Finally, anxiolytics such as benzodiazepines may be effective for the acute reduction of symptoms while waiting for the onset of action of SSRIs or for the management of uncontrollable anxiety in the acute phase of behavioral treatments. However, benzodiazepines carry the risks of sedation, dependence, and misuse, and therefore should be used sparingly and limited to short-term use.

PSYCHOSOCIAL TREATMENT

Nonpharmacologic treatments, including cognitive behavioral therapy (CBT) and family therapy, are essential for the treatment of SAD. Cognitive behavioral therapy for SAD involves psychoeducation, cognitive restructuring, exposure techniques, and learning relaxation techniques to lower anxiety. Cognitive restructuring is aimed at helping the child identify and replace unhelpful thoughts about separation with more adaptive ones. For example, a child with SAD might have the repetitive thought: "Something bad will happen to my mom if I go to school." Cognitive techniques help the child examine the likelihood of an untoward event occurring and reframing the thought in a more positive way. Exposure techniques include gradually increasing the amount of time a child is expected to be away from their parents. For example, a child who can only sleep in the same bed as her mother might start by having her mother sit next to her in her own bed for gradually decreasing periods of time, followed by her mother sitting outside of her room while she falls asleep, and so on. Finally, it can be helpful to teach the child to identify signs and symptoms of anxiety and use relaxation techniques such as deep breathing to self-soothe.

For childhood SAD, family therapy is another important intervention. Parents should be offered psychoeducation about the nature of the diagnosis and its comorbidities, as well as coaching on how to help their child manage their anxiety. Since certain parental behaviors may be linked to the diagnosis, such as enabling secondary gain from school refusal (e.g., allowing the child to watch television or play videogames at home when they avoid school), parent training can help identify and change these behaviors.

Since school refusal is very common among children and adolescents with SAD, a comprehensive treatment plan should involve the child's school. School refusal, regardless of the cause, is extremely problematic for children and adolescents, leading to academic underachievement and difficulty maintaining peer relationships. Furthermore, the longer a child is away from school, the more challenging it will be to return. Referral to a partial hospital program may be necessary for more intensive treatment to facilitate rapid school re-entry. Children with school refusal will likely require educational accommodations that can be implemented either through a Section 504 Plan or an Individualized Education Program (IEP). Home schooling is generally not recommended, as this can reinforce the child's avoidance of school. Strategies that may be helpful in addressing school refusal include developing and implementing a behavioral plan that rewards the child for school attendance, ensuring that a child can access and utilize relaxation techniques at school, and scheduled meetings with a trusted staff member when they arrive at school to ease the transition.

Navigating a new diagnosis in a child can be challenging for families. Therefore, it is essential to distribute resources that can inform and guide parents on how to best support their child. The American Academy of Child and Adolescent Psychiatry (AACAP) website has an Anxiety Disorders Resource Center, which offers valuable information for families of children with anxiety disorders (https://www.aacap.org/AACAP/Families_and_ Youth/Resource_Centers/Anxiety_Disorder_Resource_Center/Home. aspx).

KEY POINTS TO REMEMBER

- Separation anxiety disorder is a disorder of both childhood and adulthood.
- The predominant fear in SAD is that of separation from a significant attachment figure.
- Cognitive behavioral therapy is the initial treatment of choice for SAD.
- Pharmacotherapy can be utilized as an adjunct to behavioral or psychotherapeutic interventions.

Further Reading

Carmassi C, Gesi C, Massimetti E, et al. Separation anxiety disorder in the DSM-5 era. *J Psychopathol* 2015;21:365–371.

Ehrenreich JT, Santucci LC, Weiner CL. Separation anxiety disorder in youth: Phenomenology, assessment, and treatment. *Psicol Conductual* 2008;16(3):389–412.

Kirsten LT, Grenyer BF, Wagner R, et al. Impact of separation anxiety on psychotherapy outcomes for adults with anxiety disorders. *Counsel Psychother Res* 2008;8:36–42.

Masi G, Mucci M, Millepiedi S. Separation anxiety disorder in children and adolescents. *Mol Diag Ther* 2001;15:93–104.

13 Worries about being embarrassed in front of classmates

Mila N. Grossman

A 12-year-old boy presents to his pediatrician. His parents report that they are worried about his school performance and ability to socialize with peers. During one-on-one evaluation, the patient appears anxious and guarded. He responds to questions with mostly one-word answers and appears to be blushing. Physical examination is notable for sweaty palms and tachycardia but is otherwise unremarkable. A discussion with the patient's parents reveals that he has recently been trying to avoid school, especially on days when he is scheduled to give a presentation. In addition, the patient has become resistant to attending peers' birthday parties. Furthermore, teachers have raised the concern that he often eats lunch alone and does not interact with other students at recess. He has close relationships with his siblings and cousins. When his parents talk to him about these issues, he voices concern that his peers think he is "stupid" and that he will be ridiculed.

What Do You Do Now?

The patient is suffering from social anxiety disorder (SAD), characterized by excessive anxiety about social situations and fear of being scrutinized by others. The symptoms are impacting his ability to function in multiple domains, including interfering with his academic performance and ability to develop relationships with peers. Close monitoring and treatment will be necessary to prevent worsening of the symptoms and further impact on his functioning. If left untreated, SAD can lead to poor academic performance and higher rates of school dropout in addition to problems forming social and romantic relationships. Some patients may turn to using substances to relieve symptoms of SAD.

EPIDEMIOLOGY

Social anxiety disorder is quite common among children and adolescents. Approximately 6% of children and 12% of adolescents meet criteria for SAD. Symptoms of SAD can manifest as early as five years of age and the symptoms often peak in severity around the age of 12 years. The median age of onset for SAD is 13 years, and 75% of all affected individuals experience symptom onset between ages eight and 15 years. The typical age of onset in the adolescent period coincides with a time in which an individual's peer group is becoming increasingly important. Social anxiety disorder can interfere with an individual's ability to become more autonomous from their family unit and, if not treated, can have long-term sequelae affecting one's ability to function in social, academic, and professional settings. Prior to puberty, rates of SAD are relatively equal among genders; however, girls are more commonly affected than boys after puberty.

Risk factors for SAD in children and adolescents include a history of shyness or social inhibition in addition to exposure to adversity and childhood trauma. Furthermore, children and adolescents with a family history of SAD, particularly first-degree relatives, are at increased risk. The development of SAD symptoms may occur insidiously or in response to a triggering event such as an episode of bullying or being teased after a performance.

SIGNS AND SYMPTOMS

According to the *Diagnostic and Statistical Manual of Mental Disorders*, Fifth Edition (DSM-5), SAD is characterized by marked fear or anxiety about one or more social situations in which the individual is exposed to possible scrutiny by others. Examples of social situations include meeting unfamiliar people, being observed (e.g., eating or drinking), and performing in front of others (e.g., giving a speech). To meet criteria for the disorder, social situations must almost always provoke fear or anxiety, and the fear or anxiety must be out of proportion to the actual threat posed by the social situation. The individual fears that they will act in a way or show anxiety symptoms that will be negatively evaluated. Examples of negative evaluation include those that lead to feelings of humiliation, embarrassment, or rejection by others. As a result, individuals with SAD avoid social situations or endure them with intense fear or anxiety. The symptoms must be persistent, typically lasting for at least six months, and cause significant distress or impairment in the individual's ability to function. Symptoms cannot be the result of another medical condition, be attributable to the effects of medication or substance use, or be better explained by another psychiatric disorder.

The DSM-5 uses a specifier of "performance only" to characterize individuals who only experience the fear or anxiety when speaking or performing in public. Individuals with "performance only" SAD primarily experience functional impairment in school or professional settings.

Children and adolescents with SAD may present differently than adults do. For children and adolescents to meet the diagnostic criteria, the symptoms described previously must occur in the presence of peers rather than just adults. Furthermore, children may express fear or anxiety through crying, freezing, or clinging.

ASSESSMENT

The assessment of SAD begins with a comprehensive psychiatric interview to identify symptoms of social anxiety and their overall impact on the patient's functioning. Pediatricians often perform this initial evaluation. It is important to ask how the child is developing socially and inquire if the patient exhibits any reluctance or anxiety about going to school or attending social events. If the patient experiences fear or anxiety related to social situations, it is necessary to clarify if the symptoms are limited to a specific setting, such as performing in front of others, or if the symptoms are present in most social situations. Collateral information from family members, caregivers, and teachers is also helpful in establishing a diagnosis. The Severity Measure for Social Anxiety Disorder (Social Phobia)—Child Age 11–17 years is a 10-item screening tool that can be used to assess the severity of symptoms of SAD in children and adolescents. The questionnaire can be helpful in establishing a diagnosis and can also be used to track symptoms over time. In addition, the Pediatric Anxiety Rating Scale (PARS) is a 50-item tool used to assess symptoms of multiple anxiety disorders including generalized anxiety disorder (GAD), separation anxiety disorder, and SAD in children.

The mental status examination findings may include a shy-appearing individual who is difficult to engage in conversation. The individual may display limited eye contact and exhibit physical symptoms consistent with anxiety including blushing, diaphoresis, or shaking.

When evaluating for SAD, one should consider a broad differential diagnosis. First and foremost, it is necessary to rule out normative shyness, which is a common personality trait that in and of itself does not have a significant impact on one's ability to function. Other diagnoses to consider include agoraphobia, panic disorder, GAD, separation anxiety disorder, specific phobias, and selective mutism. When considering these alternative diagnoses, it is important to remember that the core symptom of SAD is the fear of scrutiny or negative evaluation by others. In contrast, patients with agoraphobia may avoid social situations due to fear of inability to escape a crowded event, while individuals with separation anxiety disorder may avoid social situations due to concern about being separated from an attachment figure. Furthermore, it is important to screen for common comorbid psychiatric disorders including other anxiety disorders (e.g., GAD, specific phobias), major depressive disorder, substance use disorders, and oppositional defiant disorder.

The initial assessment and diagnosis are often made by the patient's primary care physician; however, in situations when the diagnosis is not clear, symptoms are severe, or there is substantial psychiatric comorbidity, the patient should be referred to a psychiatrist or other behavioral health specialist for further evaluation and treatment.

BIOLOGICAL TREATMENT

Once the diagnosis of SAD is made, it is important to assess the severity of the illness and consider different treatment options. Medications can be utilized to help alleviate symptoms of SAD and are oftentimes most helpful when prescribed in conjunction with behavioral therapy. Selective serotonin reuptake inhibitors (SSRIs) and serotonin norepinephrine reuptake inhibitors (SNRIs) are first-line medication treatment options for children and adolescents with SAD. In particular, randomized controlled trials have shown that fluoxetine, paroxetine, and venlafaxine are effective in reducing symptoms of SAD in children and adolescents. Selective serotonin reuptake inhibitors and SNRIs work to increase the level of the neurotransmitters serotonin and serotonin plus norepinephrine, respectively. These medications typically take at least four to six weeks to take full effect, and common side effects include nausea, headaches, anxiety, and behavioral activation. There is a Food and Drug Administration (FDA) black-box warning for SSRIs and SNRIs regarding an increased risk of suicidal ideation and behavior in children and adolescents. As such, close monitoring for the emergence of adverse effects, particularly suicidality and behavioral activation, is imperative.

Benzodiazepines have a limited role in the treatment of pediatric SAD. Despite their rapid anxiolytic effects, this class of medications should largely be avoided in children and adolescents due to the range of potential adverse effects. Common side effects include drowsiness and the potential for behavioral activation. In addition, benzodiazepine use can lead to dependence and nonmedical use.

Beta-blockers, such as propranolol, are often utilized for performance-related social anxiety in adults. Beta-blockers can reduce physical symptoms associated with anxiety such as palpitations, sweating, and tremor. The evidence for the use of beta-blockers for SAD in children and adolescents is currently insufficient.

PSYCHOSOCIAL TREATMENT

Psychotherapy alone or in combination with medication therapy has been proven to be effective for the treatment of pediatric SAD. The most well-studied behavioral therapies are cognitive behavioral therapy (CBT) and social effectiveness therapy for children. Cognitive behavioral therapy works by teaching the child to examine and challenge their recurrent, maladaptive thoughts to reduce anxiety. Gradual exposure to social situations is another core component of CBT for SAD. Social effectiveness therapy for children is a 12-week, comprehensive behavioral treatment program that combines individual exposure therapy, group-based social skills training, and peer sessions to target pediatric SAD.

The American Academy of Child and Adolescent Psychiatry (AACAP) has published an Anxiety Disorders: Parents' Medication Guide, which can be used as a tool to provide psychoeducation about SAD, the prognosis, and treatment course (https://www.aacap.org/App_Themes/AACAP/docs/resource_centers/resources/med_guides/anxiety-parents-medication-guide.pdf).

KEY POINTS TO REMEMBER

- Social anxiety disorder affects approximately 12% of adolescents in the United States and the median age of onset is 13 years.
- To meet diagnostic criteria for SAD, children and adolescents must display symptoms of social anxiety in the presence of peers and adults.
- While the prevalence of pediatric SAD is quite high, less than 20% of affected patients receive adequate treatment.
- If not treated, SAD can have long-term effects on individuals' academic performance, professional success, and interpersonal relationships.
- Treatment for SAD in children and adolescents includes both behavioral therapy and medication therapy.

Further Reading

Beidel DC, Turner SM, Sallee FR, et al. SET-C versus fluoxetine in the treatment of childhood social phobia. *J Am Acad Child Adolesc Psychiatry* 2007;46(12):1622–1632.

Merikangas KR, He JP, Burstein M, et al. Lifetime prevalence of mental disorders in U.S. adolescents: Results from the national comorbidity survey replication— adolescent supplement (NCS-A). *J Am Acad Child Adolesc Psychiatry* 2010;49(10):980–989.

Patel DR, Feucht C, Brown K, et al. Pharmacological treatment of anxiety disorders in children and adolescents: A review for practitioners. *Transl Pediatr* 2018;7(1):23–35.

Silverman WK, Pina AA, Viswesvaran C. Evidence-based psychosocial treatments for phobic and anxiety disorders in children and adolescents. *J Clin Child Adolesc Psychol* 2008;37(1):105–130.

14 Recurrent episodes of intense fear, shortness of breath, racing heart, and sweating

Christina L. Macenski

A 17-year-old girl presents to her pediatrician with her father who reported she started refusing to go to school or swim practice three months previously. When interviewed alone, the patient stated, "I'm so scared to leave the house, my family would never understand." She reported experiencing spontaneous episodes of intense fear with shortness of breath, the sensation her heart is racing, nausea, and sweating that cause her to feel as if she is losing control. The symptoms peak in intensity within a few minutes and last for between 10 and 15 minutes. These episodes occur without a clear trigger. She fears she will be made fun of if an episode occurs at school. She started avoiding swim practices when increased heart rate reminded her of the episodes. Her medical workup, including thyroid function studies and electrocardiogram, are all within normal limits. She denies symptoms of depression and substance use including alcohol, illicit drugs, or caffeine.

What Do You Do Now?

The patient is suffering from panic disorder, an anxiety disorder characterized by recurrent and unexpected panic attacks causing fear of future attacks or a significant maladaptive change in behavior relating to them. If left untreated, panic disorder tends to be chronic in nature, but can also wax and wane with periods of exacerbation and remission. Spontaneous sustained remission without relapse is rare, suggesting that early engagement in treatment may benefit a patient's functional status and quality of life.

EPIDEMIOLOGY

The lifetime prevalence of panic disorder in adolescents aged 13 to 18 years has been estimated at 2.3%. Prevalence rates gradually increase during adolescence and peak during early adulthood, with a median age of onset between 20 and 24 years of age. The 12-month prevalence rate of panic disorder in adolescents and adults combined is about 2% to 3%. Panic disorder is significantly less common in children under the age of 14 years, with a prevalence of less than 0.4%. Panic disorder is twice as common in females as in males. Risk factors for the development of panic disorder at any age include low mood, anxiety, a history of childhood abuse, smoking, respiratory illness (such as asthma), genetic susceptibility, and parental mood or anxiety disorders. Psychiatric comorbidity with other anxiety disorders, major depressive disorder, and bipolar disorder is common. Panic attacks often first develop during a major depressive episode or during the course of separation anxiety disorder.

SIGNS AND SYMPTOMS

According to the *Diagnostic and Statistical Manual of Mental Disorders*, Fifth Edition (DSM-5), panic disorder is characterized by recurrent, unexpected panic attacks followed by one month or longer of at least one of (1) persistent concern or worry about future attacks or their consequences (e.g., losing control, having a heart attack, "going crazy") and (2) a significant maladaptive change in behavior related to the attacks (e.g., avoidance of unfamiliar situations or activities that may reproduce some symptoms of panic such as exercise). A panic attack is defined as an abrupt surge of intense fear or discomfort that reaches a peak within minutes, with four or more of the following symptoms: palpitations, pounding heart, or increased heart rate; sweating; trembling or shaking; shortness of breath; sensation of choking; chest pain or discomfort; nausea or abdominal distress; dizziness or lightheadedness; sensations of chills or heat; paresthesias; derealization (feelings of unreality) or depersonalization (being detached from oneself); fear of losing control or "going crazy"; and fear of dying. The disturbance must not be attributable to substance use or another medical condition or be better explained by another mental disorder.

Panic disorder can occur with or without agoraphobia, a marked fear or anxiety about two or more of the following situations: using public transportation, being in open spaces, being in enclosed spaces, being in a crowd or standing in line, and being outside of the home alone. The fear is due to thoughts that escape might be difficult or help might not be available in the event of developing panic-like or other embarrassing symptoms. To meet criteria for agoraphobia (which is diagnosed irrespective of the presence of panic disorder), the fear, anxiety, or avoidance must last for six months or longer.

Features of panic disorder that are more common in adolescents compared to adults include less worry about additional panic attacks and decreased willingness to openly discuss their symptoms. Compared to adults, youth with panic disorder have increased focus on the physical symptoms of panic and decreased focus on the cognitions associated with panic disorder. Overall, though, the clinical features of adolescent-onset panic disorder are quite similar to adult-onset presentations.

ASSESSMENT

Although panic disorder is a clinical diagnosis, it is important to obtain laboratory tests to rule out medical conditions that mimic panic disorder. A thorough history from both the patient and caregiver is the crux of an effective evaluation and should include detailed information about the panic attacks (such as typical symptoms, frequency, duration, level of distress), potential triggers (some of which may not be immediately recognized by the patient), anxiety symptoms in between panic attacks, past medical and psychiatric history, substance use history (including caffeine intake), medications, history of major life events, social history, and family history. An exploration of the patient's understanding or insight into their illness along with psychosocial stressors and supports is also important. It is important to establish a strong therapeutic alliance since the symptoms of panic disorder can be embarrassing for adolescents to discuss.

The mental status examination is often normal in patients with panic disorder unless a panic attack occurs during the assessment. If so, the adolescent may appear confused or fearful, with either normal or rapid speech, anxious mood with congruent affect, logical and linear thought processes, and thought content focused on the consequences of the panic attack; suicidal ideation may be present, and insight/judgment during a panic attack can range from poor to good. The cognitive examination is expected to be normal for age and educational level. If the patient is not experiencing a panic attack during the assessment, the patient may describe an anxious mood or other abnormalities depending on whether psychiatric comorbidities are present. Because there can be symptom overlap among different anxiety disorders, it may be useful to use a standardized semistructured interview tool such as the Anxiety Disorders Interview Schedule: Child and Parent Versions (ADIS-CP) to differentiate among them. The ADIS-CP can assess for all of the anxiety disorders listed in the DSM-5 and is considered the gold standard for assessment. The use of this scale may be limited in clinical practice, as it is not open access due to copyright restrictions.

All patients with suspected panic disorder should undergo a complete physical examination with a laboratory workup that includes a complete blood count, serum electrolytes, blood glucose level, hemoglobin A1c, thyroid-stimulating hormone, urine toxicology, and electrocardiogram. In older adults, cardiac enzymes and D-dimer to rule out acute coronary syndromes and pulmonary embolism, respectively, are also reasonable in at-risk patients but have limited utility in children and adolescents who are otherwise medically healthy. Additional workup can be considered based on the clinical presentation and results of the preliminary workup.

The differential diagnosis for panic disorder is broad and includes psychiatric disorders including somatic symptom disorder, illness anxiety disorder, and substance use disorders (e.g., stimulants, caffeine), as well as medical conditions such as hyperthyroidism, pheochromocytoma, arrhythmias, asthma, seizure disorders, and intoxication. Mood and other anxiety disorders are highly comorbid with panic disorder and all patients should be screened for psychiatric comorbidity.

LEVEL OF CARE

Most patients diagnosed with panic disorder are managed in the outpatient setting. However, there may be certain circumstances that necessitate a higher level of care such as a partial hospital program, inpatient hospitalization, or home visits. Hospitalization can be considered when acute suicidality or substance use requires close monitoring. Rarely, inpatient hospitalization may be warranted when panic disorder is severe or associated with agoraphobia or when outpatient management fails. Home visits or telemedicine appointments may be an option when agoraphobia limits the patient's ability to leave the house.

BIOLOGICAL TREATMENT

There are several Food and Drug Administration (FDA)-approved medications to treat panic disorder in adults including the selective serotonin reuptake inhibitors (SSRIs) fluoxetine, paroxetine, and sertraline; the serotonin norepinephrine reuptake inhibitor (SNRI) venlafaxine; and the benzodiazepines alprazolam and clonazepam. It should be noted there are no FDA-approved medications for panic disorder in children and adolescents; however, SSRIs and SNRIs are commonly used first-line medications in child and adolescent anxiety disorders. Psychopharmacologic treatment is recommended when panic disorder symptoms are moderate to severe or when there are significant barriers to accessing psychotherapy, including symptom severity that limits participation and geographic barriers to accessing care.

Second-line medications for panic disorder in children and adolescents include tricyclic antidepressants (TCAs) and benzodiazepines. While TCAs are a reasonable alternative to SSRIs and SNRIs, the increased side effect and toxicity profile must be considered. Benzodiazepines may be useful as a short-term adjunctive treatment. Benzodiazepines are contraindicated in patients with substance use disorders and can cause side effects such as sedation, cognitive impairment, dependence, and disinhibition.

Children and adolescents with panic disorder may be more sensitive to the physical side effects of medications, which can be particularly problematic in adolescents who are already at high risk for nonadherence. Medications often need to be started at low dosages and increased gradually. Preemptive discussion about side effects and the safety profile of medications prior to prescribing is important. It is also important to educate families and patients about the FDA black-box warning concerning the potential for increased suicidality associated with SSRIs and SNRIs.

Expert consensus suggests that effective pharmacotherapy for panic disorder be continued for at least one year after attaining remission. Decisions about when and how to discontinue medications should follow a collaborative discussion involving the clinician, patient, and caregiver, with particular attention to the possibility of recurrence of panic disorder symptoms and withdrawal side effects if the medication is discontinued. It is prudent to taper the medication gradually over weeks to months and to monitor for symptom recurrence, with prompt medication reinitiation if recurrence occurs and is distressing.

PSYCHOSOCIAL TREATMENT

Psychoeducation about the symptoms, course, prognosis, and treatment options for panic disorder is the first step in treatment. The American Academy of Child and Adolescent Psychiatry (AACAP) has published a Facts for Families article with helpful information for parents (https://www.aacap.org/App_Themes/AACAP/docs/facts_for_families/50_panic_disorder_in_children_and_adolescents.pdf). The treatment goals for panic disorder are to decrease functional impairment and increase quality of life. This can be accomplished with different types of therapy including cognitive behavioral therapy (CBT), psychodynamic psychotherapy, and family therapy. Cognitive behavioral therapy has the strongest evidence for the treatment of panic disorder and is considered a first-line psychotherapy option. There are five major components of CBT for anxiety disorders: psychoeducation, somatic management skills training, cognitive restructuring, exposure exercises, and relapse prevention. Booster sessions may be offered to decrease the risk of relapse.

Cognitive behavioral therapy interventions specific to panic disorder include interoceptive exposures (inducing physical sensations of a panic attack under controlled conditions) and education about the sympathetic nervous system. Examples of interoceptive exposures include breathing quickly through a straw to induce hyperventilation, intense exercise to increase heart rate, and spinning in a chair to cause dizziness. By practicing these exposures, the patient learns to tolerate and manage distress associated with the physical symptoms of panic. The patient also learns that the symptoms of panic are not dangerous. Education about the sympathetic nervous system can include information about the physiological processes that lead to the physical sensations of a panic attack. Family therapy may also be useful when parenting styles or parent-child interactions serve to reinforce or maintain the symptoms of panic disorder but should not be the sole psychotherapeutic intervention. While there is robust clinical experience with psychodynamic psychotherapy for the treatment of anxiety disorders, formal research is limited, and more data is needed prior to drawing conclusions about efficacy. The central themes of panic-focused psychodynamic therapy for adolescents with panic disorder may include identifying core conflicts such as those relating to separation and dependency.

KEY POINTS TO REMEMBER

- Panic disorder is an anxiety disorder characterized by recurrent, unexpected panic attacks that cause persistent worry/concern about future attacks or maladaptive behavioral changes related to the attacks.
- Panic attacks are defined as an abrupt onset of fear or discomfort that peaks within minutes and is associated with at least four symptoms defined by the DSM-5. Symptoms include palpitations, sweating, shaking, shortness of breath, chest pain, abdominal discomfort, dizziness, lightheadedness, paresthesias, derealization, depersonalization, or fear of dying/losing control.
- Panic disorder is a clinical diagnosis, although medical causes of panic attacks must be excluded.

- Biological treatments include SSRIs, SNRIs, TCAs, and time-limited use of benzodiazepines. Children and adolescents with panic disorder may be particularly sensitive to medication side effects.
- Cognitive behavioral therapy is considered the gold standard therapy intervention for panic disorder.

Further Reading

Connolly SD, Bernstein GA. Practice parameter for the assessment and treatment of children and adolescents with anxiety disorders. *J Am Acad Child Adolesc Psychiatry* 2007;46(2):267–283.

Freidl EK, Stroeh OM, Elkins RM, et al. Assessment and treatment of anxiety among children and adolescents. *Focus* 2017;15(2):144–156.

Hella B, Bernstein GA. Panic disorder and school refusal. *Child Adolesc Psychiatr Clin* 2012;21(3):593–606.

Wang Z, Whiteside SP, Sim L, et al. Comparative effectiveness and safety of cognitive behavioral therapy and pharmacotherapy for childhood anxiety disorders: A systematic review and meta-analysis. *JAMA Pediatr* 2017;171(11):1049–1056.

15 Excessive, uncontrollable worries

Joseph A. Pereira

A 12-year-old girl presents for an outpatient psychiatric evaluation for excessive anxiety. She is accompanied by her mother, who expresses concern that her daughter is frequently worrying about her grades, the safety of her family members, and various other concerns throughout the day. Her teachers have mentioned that she also seems very anxious at school, for example, frequently asking for help when she already understands the assignment.

On psychiatric assessment, the patient is restless and tense. She confirms that she worries about many things throughout the day, including her academic performance, what people think about her, her future, and whether her parents are safe. On multiple occasions, she interrupts the interview to ask if her mother is sure that she locked the car door, as she is fearful someone might steal the music player she left inside. Her mother notes that her excessive worry has been consistent since she was old enough to articulate her worries. She has no significant medical conditions and her family history is positive for an "anxiety disorder" in her maternal aunt and grandmother.

What Do You Do Now?

The patient's presentation is consistent with generalized anxiety disorder (GAD). Generalized anxiety disorder is characterized by excessive and uncontrollable worry that occurs on most days for at least six months. The worry is present in multiple settings, with concerns about a wide range of issues. Many factors contribute to the development of GAD, including biological, psychological, and social influences. The recognition and treatment of GAD is imperative, as uncontrolled GAD can lead to a high use of medical services and functional impairment.

EPIDEMIOLOGY

Although the prevalence of GAD increases with age, pediatric-onset GAD generally begins around the age of seven years. The prevalence ranges from 3% to 6% in children and adolescents. In adults, GAD is twice as common in females than in males, but the gender distribution is more equal in youth. A behaviorally inhibited temperament, insecure attachment style, high levels of parental discipline, adverse childhood experiences, lack of prosocial school behavior, inattention, and anxious parental modeling have all been cited as risk factors for developing GAD.

Generalized anxiety disorder is a chronic condition, with symptoms waxing and waning throughout one's lifetime. Full remission rates are low, but symptoms can be managed with a combination of psychotherapy and pharmacology. The diagnosis of GAD in childhood is associated with greater symptom severity, heritability, functional impairment, and comorbidity. Common comorbid conditions include major depressive disorder (MDD) and other anxiety disorders.

SIGNS AND SYMPTOMS

According to the *Diagnostic and Statistical Manual of Mental Disorders*, Fifth Edition (DSM-5), GAD is characterized by excessive anxiety and worry that occurs more days than not for at least six months. The worry is present across different settings and is difficult to control. In children and adolescents, one of the following symptoms must be exhibited more days than not over a six-month period: restless or feeling keyed up or on edge, being easily fatigued, difficulty concentrating or mind going blank, irritability, muscle tension, or sleep disturbance. This differs from the adult diagnosis of GAD, which requires at least three of these symptoms to be present. The symptoms associated with GAD must cause impairment in the individual's life. Finally, the effects of a substance or another condition should not better explain the symptoms.

Several behavioral symptoms are commonly associated with GAD in children. These may include crying episodes, temper tantrums, and increased irritability. Younger children may also develop hair pulling and nail biting as a consequence of uncontrolled anxiety. Compared to adults with GAD, children and adolescents also more commonly report somatic complaints. These may include gastrointestinal upset (e.g., stomachaches, nausea, vomiting), headaches, and diaphoresis.

ASSESSMENT

Biological, psychological, and social approaches should be used when assessing a child or adolescent for GAD. It is important to determine the history of onset and evolution of anxiety symptoms, including when, where, how often, and for how long the symptoms last. When possible, information should be collected from the patient, caregiver(s), school, and other appropriate collateral sources. Young children, in particular, may have difficulty communicating their experience of anxiety, while older children are often more accurate than their caregivers in reporting such symptoms. A developmental approach should be taken when assessing if individuals meet DSM-5 criteria for GAD, as it is important to differentiate between excessive worry and developmentally normal fears.

Features of the mental status examination consistent with GAD may include evidence of restlessness, tense posture, tremor, diaphoresis, and anxious ruminations. Rating scales can be used to better characterize the symptomatology of GAD and determine the level of severity. Measures such as the Behavior Assessment System for Children, Second Edition (BASC-2), include self-report, caregiver report, teacher report, and clinician report to provide a comprehensive overview of a child's behavioral issues. Additional measures include the Screen for Child Anxiety Related Disorders (SCARED), which includes both child and caregiver reports.

Biological Assessment

A complete medical history and physical examination should be completed as part of the clinical evaluation for GAD, with particular attention to medical conditions that may mimic its symptomatology. These include hyperthyroidism, hypoglycemia, asthma, pheochromocytoma, substance withdrawal/intoxication, and medication side effects (e.g., stimulant medications). Laboratory tests can be a helpful adjunct in assessing these conditions (e.g., thyroid function tests, glucose levels, urine toxicology screen). The clinical evaluation should also include a thorough family psychiatric history, as anxiety disorders show moderate to strong heritability. Inquiry and documentation of somatic symptoms during the initial evaluation can help clinicians track their presentation and help the child and caregiver understand their relationship with GAD.

Psychological Assessment

A detailed developmental history should be obtained, with particular attention to the child's temperament and attachment style. Fears should be evaluated to determine if they are developmentally appropriate rather than pathological. Developmentally normal fears are transient and nonimpairing and respond to reassurance. Common developmentally normal fears include fear of the dark, monsters, ghosts, and burglars. Inquiry into the feelings, thoughts, and behaviors of children and adolescents with suspected GAD is recommended. Their feelings are marked by self-consciousness and persistent worry even when there is no realistic cause for concern. They may have cognitive distortions and believe that anything other than perfection is a failure, focusing on mistakes and negative consequences rather than successes. Children with GAD also often have difficulty tolerating uncertainty. Behaviorally, they may be observed to require frequent reassurance from others, display traits of perfectionism, and exhibit self-criticism. Learned behaviors, such as mimicking an anxious parent, may contribute to GAD and can be assessed for through direct observation of the caregiver-child interaction or through inquiry.

Social Assessment

When applicable, information about a child's or adolescent's anxiety symptoms should be gathered from multiple sources, including teachers and caregivers. During this evaluation, investigation into social stressors and negative life events can help determine critical contributors to the symptomatology. A school history is particularly important, as teachers can often readily recognize if a child's anxiety is impairing their academic or social functioning relative to same-age peers. Assessment of peer relationships should focus on experiences of bullying, rejection, or neglect. Children and adolescents with GAD often exhibit unfounded persistent worry about interpersonal relationships and have negative self-evaluation in social situations.

Differential Diagnosis

Generalized anxiety disorder is associated with several comorbid psychiatric disorders. These conditions can be misdiagnosed as GAD and should therefore be considered in the differential diagnosis. In particular, other anxiety disorders, such as separation anxiety disorder, social anxiety disorder, panic disorder, or specific phobias, are all highly comorbid with but also often misdiagnosed as GAD. These can be differentiated on the basis of the content of the fear. Importantly, children and adolescents with GAD have worries about a wide range of topics. Mood disorders, particularly MDD, also tend to be comorbid with GAD and should be assessed through clinical evaluation. Attention-deficit/hyperactivity disorder is another common comorbid condition that should be included in the differential diagnosis. It is characterized by excessive inattention and behaving "as if driven by a motor," rather than excessive worry. Notably, children with GAD can have difficulty concentrating due to excessive worrying, but when they are not anxious, their attention and concentration should be intact. Finally, the presence of somatic symptoms should prompt the consideration of a nonpsychiatric etiology.

BIOLOGICAL TREATMENT

Pharmacotherapy should not be used as the sole treatment for GAD, but rather as an adjunct to psychotherapy. When deciding whether to initiate pharmacotherapy, factors to consider include the child's response to psychotherapy alone, the severity of the anxiety symptoms as they pertain to the level of functioning, and the age of the child (medications are often less effective and less well tolerated in younger children). There is evidence to suggest that medication therapy in combination with psychotherapy is more effective than either treatment alone.

Selective serotonin reuptake inhibitors (SSRIs) and serotonin norepinephrine reuptake inhibitors (SNRIs) are considered first-line medications for the treatment of GAD. Currently, duloxetine is the only drug with Food and Drug Administration (FDA) approval for treating pediatric GAD. Since there is no evidence that one SSRI or SNRI is more effective than another, the medication's tolerability, side effect profile, and formulation may be used to select a starting medication. If the first medication is ineffective, a trial of another SSRI or SNRI is recommended. Both SSRIs and SNRIs are generally well tolerated and are relatively low risk for toxicity with overdose. Important side effects to monitor for include transient anxiety or agitation during the initiation or uptitration of the medication. All SSRIs and SNRIs carry an FDA black-box warning indicating that they may be associated with increased suicidality. Although the benefits of using an SSRI or SNRI likely outweigh the risks when treating pediatric depressive and anxiety disorders, the emergence of suicidal thoughts should be monitored for with caution. Guidelines suggest maintenance of a therapeutic dose of the medication for one year from symptom remission; however, many patients with anxiety disorders benefit from longer-term treatment with medication. If the decision is made to taper the medication, it should be decreased during a low-stress time with close monitoring for recurrence of symptoms.

Second-line or adjunctive classes of medication that can be used in refractory or severe cases of GAD include alpha$_2$ adrenergic agonist medications (clonidine or guanfacine), buspirone (a serotonin partial agonist), or second-generation antipsychotics.

PSYCHOLOGICAL TREATMENT

Cognitive behavioral therapy (CBT) is the most evidence-based psychotherapy for GAD. Cognitive behavioral therapy techniques may vary for each child depending on their presenting symptoms but generally include cognitive restructuring, problem-solving techniques, and relaxation exercises. Cognitive restructuring is fundamental, as it leads to more adaptive behaviors through the reconstruction of fear-sustaining thoughts. For younger children (seven years and younger), CBT should be modified to include increased parental involvement, exposure exercises through games, and more immediate positive reinforcement. In general, CBT is most effective when the skills are practiced in several settings, including at home and at school.

Parent-child interventions are imperative, as child-only interventions may not adequately address contributing factors such as insecure attachment, caregiver anxiety, and controlling parental styles. Parental involvement in their child's therapy or initiation of their own individual therapy can lead to a deeper understanding of their child's condition. This can promote greater encouragement of the child's independence, improved communication skills, and reduced parental anxiety. In addition, family therapy can be effective in mitigating dysfunctional family dynamics that promote anxiety, while supporting effective behaviors. Psychoeducation can further deepen caregivers' understanding of GAD. The American Academy of Child and Adolescent Psychiatry (AACAP) has published a Facts for Families article on anxiety (https://www.aacap.org/ AACAP/Families_and_Youth/Facts_for_Families/FFF-Guide/The-Anxious-Child-047.aspx), which can be distributed to parents.

Parent guidance for GAD can be included to decrease parental accommodation of a child's anxiety and may be used as an alternative to CBT, particularly for younger children or children who cannot engage in CBT treatment. Parental accommodation refers to ways in which parents accommodate the child's symptoms of anxiety, such as providing reassurance, allowing children to avoid feared stimuli, and modifying family routines. Although accommodation of anxiety reduces fear in the short term, it results in continued dependence on the parent to regulate anxiety and contributes to the maintenance of the symptoms of GAD. Parental accommodation is present in 95% of parents of anxious children and is associated with more severe anxiety symptoms. Parent-based treatment that focuses on reducing parental accommodation behaviors in parents of children with GAD has been shown to be noninferior to CBT.

SOCIAL TREATMENT

Interventions aimed at a child's environment are important to decrease the negative social factors that may contribute to GAD and aid in the restructuring of negative cognitions centered on social situations. Clinical consultations with school personnel and others can help coordinate these efforts. Increasing peer and social supports both in and out of school can be an important way to foster adaptive social behavior without causing excessive anxiety. Academically, specific recommendations and accommodations tailored for GAD can be included in a child's Section 504 Plan or Individualized Education Program (IEP). Teachers and other school professionals should be educated on GAD and effective coping strategies.

KEY POINTS TO REMEMBER

- Generalized anxiety disorder occurs in 3% to 6% of children and adolescents with prevalence increasing with age.
- Hallmarks of GAD in children and adolescents include excessive worry and anxiety in multiple settings over at least a six-month period.
- Behavioral dysregulation and somatic symptoms may be symptoms of GAD in children and adolescents.
- An assessment of GAD should utilize a development approach with emphasis on biological, psychological, and social factors that might contribute to the symptomatology.
- Psychotherapies for GAD include CBT and parent guidance to decrease accommodating behaviors.
- Pharmacotherapy options include SSRIs and SNRIs.

Further Reading

Connolly SD, Bernstein GA, Work Group on Quality Issues. Practice parameter for the assessment and treatment of children and adolescents with anxiety disorders. *J Am Acad Child Adolesc Psychiatry* 2007;46(2):267–283.

Connolly S, Suárez L, Victor A, et al. Anxiety disorders. In: Dulcan MK, ed., *Dulcan's Textbook of Child and Adolescent Psychiatry*. Arlington, VA: American Psychiatric Association Publishing, 2016:Chapter 15.

Katzman MA, Bleau P, Blier P, et al. Canadian clinical practice guidelines for the management of anxiety, posttraumatic stress and obsessive-compulsive disorders. *BMC Psychiatry* 2014;14(S1):1–83.

Rapee RM. Anxiety disorders in children and adolescents: Nature, development, treatment and prevention. In: Rey JM, ed., *IACAPAP e-Textbook of Child and Adolescent Mental Health*. Geneva: International Association for Child and Adolescent Psychiatry and Allied Professions, 2017:Chapter F.1, 1–20.

Stein MB, Sareen J. Generalized anxiety disorder. *N Engl J Med* 2015;373(21):2059–2068.

16 A teenager who spends hours scrutinizing her skin

Kevin M. Hill

A 16-year-old female is referred for a psychiatric evaluation because of symptoms of depression and anxiety. She has become sad and worried, very isolated, avoiding going out with friends and finding excuses to miss school. Her grades have also dropped. She avoids leaving home because she is highly concerned about her "terrible acne." She spends several hours per day scrutinizing her skin in the mirror. She feels that her appearance is so "hideous" that she isolates in her room and avoids being seen in public. If she must go out, she goes to great lengths to "hide" her acne. She styles her hair so that it covers as much of her face as possible and her makeup routine takes more than an hour to complete. She has seen multiple dermatologists all of whom have seemed dismissive of her concerns. On examination, the patient has a few scattered comedones across her forehead, but otherwise her skin is clear.

What Do You Do Now?

This patient is likely suffering from body dysmorphic disorder (BDD), characterized by an impairing and distressing preoccupation with a perceived defect in appearance that either is not observable or appears slight to others. Individuals with BDD often have poor insight into their illness and the repetitive behaviors (e.g., checking, scrutinizing, comparing) they perform in response to their concerns can result in considerable distress and/or impairment. Many individuals with BDD do not seek treatment due to their embarrassment regarding the perceived flaw and lack of insight.

EPIDEMIOLOGY

The prevalence of BDD among adolescents globally ranges from 2% to 4%, with female predominance (~80%). In terms of onset, two-thirds of all patients develop BDD before the age of 18 years. The most common age of onset is 12 to 13 years. In comparison to patients who develop BDD as adults, adolescent-onset BDD is associated with a more gradual progression of symptoms, higher rates of psychiatric comorbidity, and higher rates of suicide attempts. A prior history of childhood abuse and neglect is a risk factor for developing BDD. Many adolescents with BDD seek cosmetic treatment for their perceived defect (e.g., dermatological, surgical, dental).

SIGNS AND SYMPTOMS

The *Diagnostic and Statistical Manual of Mental Disorders*, Fifth Edition (DSM-5), classifies BDD as an obsessive-compulsive and related disorder. The DSM-5 criteria for BDD include a preoccupation with one or more perceived defects or flaws in physical appearance that are not observable or appear slight to others. The individual engages in repetitive behaviors or mental acts in response to the appearance concerns. Examples of repetitive behaviors include excessive grooming, skin picking, mirror checking, or reassurance seeking. Common repetitive mental acts include comparing their appearance to others. The symptoms must be severe enough to cause significant distress and/or impair functioning.

The DSM-5 includes an insight specifier, where individuals with good or fair insight recognize that the BDD beliefs are definitely or probably not true, while individuals with poor insight believe that the beliefs are probably true. The adolescent's degree of insight, their level of conviction regarding the abnormal belief, can fluctuate over time. Insight typically worsens during periods of stress, while it typically improves transiently with reassurance. The DSM-5 also includes an additional specifier, "with muscle dysmorphia," to specify patients who are preoccupied with the idea that their body build is insufficiently muscular.

ASSESSMENT

The initial evaluation of BDD begins with a psychiatric history and mental status examination, specifically inquiring about delusional thought content related to body image preoccupations as well as repetitive behaviors. In general, an interview assessing for BDD symptomatology can be initiated with a question such as "Are you worried about the way you look?" or "Are you unhappy with how you look?" The interviewer can then inquire about whether there are any specific areas of concern, how much time the patient spends worrying about their appearance, how these concerns interfere with their daily activities (school, friends, social interactions, family), and how distressing the perceived defect is. The most common areas of concern include skin, hair, stomach, weight, and teeth. It should also be determined whether the patient has ever thought about or sought out cosmetic interventions (dermatology visits, surgical interventions, etc.) to "correct" the perceived defect.

Since many patients with BDD may be too self-conscious to report their symptoms freely, a few screening tools have been developed to aid the diagnostic evaluation. The two most widely used screening tools are the BDD version of the Yale-Brown Obsessive Compulsive Scale (BDD-YBOCS) and the Body Dysmorphic Disorder Questionnaire (BDDQ). The BDD-YBOCS, a 12-item structured assessment, is the gold standard for assessing the severity of BDD. However, it is less practical to administer in many clinical settings as it requires specialty training to administer and is a lengthier assessment. The BDDQ, a four-item assessment tool, is a reasonable alternative. It is both sensitive (94% to 100%) and specific (89% to 93%) for BDD.

Finally, the importance of a thorough suicide risk assessment cannot be overemphasized. Body dysmorphic disorder is associated with an increased risk of both suicidal ideation and suicide attempts. One study demonstrated that 81% of adolescents with BDD had a history of suicidal ideation and 44% had a history of a previous suicide attempt. The existence of a co-morbid psychiatric disorder further increases suicide risk. A suicide risk assessment should include whether the patient is experiencing urges to harm themselves, thoughts of suicide, suicide plans or preparation, access to means, history of past suicide attempts, and family history of suicides.

The differential diagnosis for BDD includes eating disorders and developmentally normal appearance concerns or clearly noticeable physical defects. While eating disorders can coexist with BDD, it is important to distinguish between these disorders. Those with BDD tend to focus on physical defects, while those with eating disorders tend to focus more on body weight and body shape. Also, while a patient with BDD may present with some weight-related concerns, they do not usually engage in markedly abnormal eating behaviors such as restricting caloric intake, binging, or purging. It is also important to distinguish BDD from the developmentally normal appearance concerns that can be common during adolescence. It can be normal for adolescents to be more focused on their physical appearance than they were as younger children. Factors that may contribute to nonpathological body image disturbance during adolescence include the normative importance of appearance during adolescence, body changes associated with puberty, emerging sexuality, and identity formation. However, an adolescent would qualify for a diagnosis of BDD if there is decreased insight regarding the physical defect, it causes a great deal of distress, and the associated repetitive behaviors are time consuming and interfere with other activities. Other common comorbid psychiatric disorders include major depressive disorder and anxiety disorders.

BIOLOGICAL TREATMENT

Extrapolating from the adult literature, the first-line class of medications for the treatment of BDD is selective serotonin reuptake inhibitors (SSRIs). Very little data examining medication treatments in youth with BDD is available; however, case series and case report data suggest that youth with BDD may also benefit from SSRIs. In adult BDD, fluoxetine and escitalopram are the two SSRIs that have been the most extensively studied.

However, it is reasonable to use any SSRI for the treatment of BDD, with the exception of citalopram (discussed later). While it is important to acknowledge the Food and Drug Administration (FDA) black-box warning regarding suicidal ideation with the use of SSRIs in adolescents, particularly in light of the association between BDD and increased suicidality, this should not preclude the use of SSRIs in youth with BDD when careful monitoring and close psychiatric follow-up are possible.

In terms of dosage, patients with BDD tend to require relatively high doses of SSRIs. For this reason, the SSRI citalopram should be excluded from treatment of BDD due to its dose-dependent cardiac side effects (QTc interval prolongation).

A relatively longer SSRI trial duration of 12 to 16 weeks is recommended to determine response, compared with SSRI trials for major depressive disorder and anxiety disorders. Providers should not discontinue treatment with a medication, labeling it "ineffective" for BDD, until the patient has been on the medication for at least 12 weeks. Of note, it is recommended that to be considered an adequate medication trial, the patient should be treated with a high dose of the SSRI (often either the highest dose tolerated or the highest dose recommended by the manufacturer) for the last two to three weeks of the treatment period. Some clinicians even exceed the maximum dose recommended by the manufacturer if the patient demonstrates a partial response. Many patients with BDD require long-term treatment with SSRIs, due to the high risk of relapse when SSRIs are discontinued. For refractory cases with a partial response to the SSRI, augmentation with buspirone, a serotonin receptor partial agonist, may be considered. Augmentation with a first- or second-generation antipsychotic is an alternative approach, particularly for patients with poor insight.

PSYCHOLOGICAL TREATMENT

The literature on psychotherapy for adolescents with BDD is limited. Single case reports have demonstrated that cognitive behavioral therapy (CBT) for adolescents with BDD is an effective psychotherapy option. In these reports, CBT has been shown to significantly improve symptoms of BDD as well as the symptoms of comorbid anxiety and depression. While the recommended frequency of therapy sessions varies among studies, once-weekly treatment is generally sufficient.

SOCIAL TREATMENT

Body dysmorphic disorder can have significant impacts on day-to-day functioning. In fact, in one case series, 85% of adolescents with BDD reported that their school performance was negatively impacted by their symptoms due to school avoidance (39%) or dropping out of school (18%). Therefore, as a provider, it is important to educate families on this matter so that they can seek education accommodations through a Section 504 Plan or Individualized Education Program (IEP).

Caring for a child with BDD can also be a significant challenge for the parent and family. Therefore, it is critical that family members actively take note of this and take measures to take care of themselves and find support for the family as well. It is important that family members offer support to the patient and encourage participation in treatment, while limiting their involvement in and accommodation of the patient's BDD rituals. The International OCD Foundation has published an article on BDD for families, which can provide helpful information for parents and caregivers (https://bdd.iocdf.org/for-families/).

KEY POINTS TO REMEMBER

- The hallmark of BDD is preoccupation with a defect in physical appearance that is either minimal or nonexistent. This preoccupation leads to repetitive behaviors that can result in distress and/or impairment in functioning.
- Body dysmorphic disorder usually begins in adolescence with a prevalence 2% to 4% of adolescents worldwide.
- Many patients do not divulge their symptoms to medical providers unless specifically asked about them due to shame and embarrassment.
- Assessment tools such as the BDDQ and the BDD-YBOCS can help aid in the diagnosis and evaluation of BDD.
- The primary treatments for BDD are SSRIs and CBT.

Further Reading

Albertini RS, Phillips KA. Thirty-three cases of body dysmorphic disorder in children and adolescents. *J Am Acad Child Adolesc Psychiatry* 1999;38(4):453–459.

Krebs G, Fernandez de la Cruz L, Mataix-Cols D. Recent advances in understanding and managing body dysmorphic disorder. *Evid Based Mental Health* 2017;20(3):71–75.

Phillips KA. Pharmacotherapy for body dysmorphic disorder. *Psychiatr Ann* 2010;40(7):325–332.

Phillips KA, Didie ER, Menard W, et al. Clinical features of body dysmorphic disorder in adolescents and adults. *Psychiatry Res* 2006;141:305–314.

Repeating, counting, and touching to prevent harm

Ivana Viani

A 17-year-old nonbinary individual is brought to the psychiatrist's office by their parents due to increasing isolation and deteriorating school performance. The patient has been spending up to five hours per day adjusting objects in their room, touching doorknobs a specific number of times, and counting to 100 prior to entering or leaving their room. The patient believes that if they fail to perform these rituals, "something really bad" will happen to their parents. The patient acknowledges this is "illogical" but explains that the rituals are very difficult to resist. When they try to resist engaging in them, they experience increasing anxiety, which is only relieved by completing the ritual. They have been engaging in these rituals for the past five years. The rituals interfere with the patient's ability to get to school on time, complete their homework, and socialize with peers.

On examination, there are no delusions, hallucinations, thoughts of harm to self or others or depressed mood.

What Do You Do Now?

This patient meets the *Diagnostic and Statistical Manual of Mental Disorders*, Fifth Edition (DSM-5), criteria for obsessive-compulsive disorder (OCD). Untreated, the condition tends to have a chronic course in about 50% of patients, with only 20% achieving full recovery spontaneously. The impact of OCD symptoms on a person's functioning can be developmentally detrimental and long-lasting, leading to poor quality of life and impaired social, academic, and occupational functioning. Early recognition and treatment are associated with improved outcomes.

EPIDEMIOLOGY

The prevalence of OCD is 1% to 3% worldwide in children and adolescents, with relatively equal incidence in both sexes, though male individuals tend to develop symptoms earlier in life. Obsessive-compulsive disorder is a relatively early-onset condition, with symptoms typically beginning between the ages of 10 and 21 years. The age of onset has a bimodal distribution, clustering around the ages of eight to 12 years (early onset) and late teens to early 20s. Early-onset OCD is associated with more severe OCD symptoms and greater treatment resistance. Risk factors for the development of OCD include a family history of OCD, childhood physical or sexual abuse, social isolation, and perinatal complications such as preterm birth, low birth weight, and high birth weight. Up to 90% of people diagnosed with OCD will meet criteria for at least one other psychiatric disorder. The most commonly co-occurring psychiatric conditions are anxiety disorders, trichotillomania, tic disorders, neurodevelopmental disorders, attention-deficit/hyperactivity disorder, major depressive disorder, and oppositional defiant disorder.

SIGNS AND SYMPTOMS

According to the DSM-5, the diagnosis of OCD requires the presence of obsessions and/or compulsions that are time-consuming (more than one hour per day) or cause clinically significant distress or impairment in functioning. Obsessions are recurrent and persistent intrusive, unwanted thoughts, urges, or images that cause marked anxiety or distress in most individuals. The individual attempts to ignore or suppress these thoughts, urges, or images, or to neutralize them with some other thought or action. Compulsions are repetitive behaviors or mental acts that an individual feels compelled to perform in response to an obsession or according to rules that must be applied rigidly. The behaviors or mental acts are aimed at preventing some dreaded event or situation but are not realistically connected with what they are designed to neutralize or prevent and are clearly excessive. Young children may not be able to articulate the aims of these behaviors or mental acts. The content of the obsessions and compulsions can be widely variable, with themes of symmetry, cleanliness/contamination, and unacceptable ideas of harm being among the most common. Examples of obsessions include worrying about germs, the feeling that things need to be "just right," worrying about bad things happening or doing something wrong, disturbing thoughts or images about hurting others, and disturbing sexual thoughts or images. Examples of compulsions include washing/cleaning; confessing, checking, or apologizing; tapping, touching, or rubbing; ordering or arranging; repeating an action until it feels "just right"; mentally checking; or repeating lucky words or numbers.

The DSM-5 includes two main specifiers for OCD: whether the disorder is tic related (current or past history of a tic disorder) and what level of insight the person possesses (good/fair, poor, or absent/delusional).

The onset of OCD symptoms is typically gradual. Children often hide rituals from adults initially, but this becomes more difficult as the symptoms progress in severity. Engaging in rituals is often suppressible, especially when the child is outside of their home. It can be more difficult to resist engaging in rituals when at home or with family members. The natural history of OCD is for the content of obsessions and compulsions to change with time and for the urge to perform compulsions to intensify without treatment.

Obsessive-compulsive disorder can be impairing due to the time-consuming nature of obsessions and compulsions. In one survey study, subjects diagnosed with OCD reported experiencing obsessions for approximately six hours per day and engaging in compulsions for over four hours per day. Children and adolescents with OCD also commonly avoid places, individuals, and situations that might trigger their symptoms.

ASSESSMENT

Many people with obsessions and/or compulsions will hide their symptoms since they are ego-dystonic and may cause shame and embarrassment. This tends to delay the diagnosis and treatment, leading to poorer outcomes. Clinicians are well advised to screen for OCD routinely.

Obsessive-compulsive disorder is diagnosed on the basis of the clinical interview and mental status examination. The most widely accepted rating scale for children and adolescents is the Children's Yale-Brown Obsessive Compulsive Scale (CY-BOCS), which is a clinician-administered questionnaire assessing both the presence and severity of obsessions and compulsions. The CY-BOCS can be used to aid in making the diagnosis and to track treatment response.

It is important to note that some repetitive or ritualistic behaviors can be developmentally normal in childhood. These behaviors must be distinguished from OCD. Compared with the compulsions that occur in the setting of an OCD diagnosis, developmentally appropriate repetitive behaviors are not overly time-consuming, do not interfere with family functioning, are enjoyable for the child to engage in, and can be skipped or modified without causing distress.

BIOLOGICAL TREATMENT

The Pediatric OCD Treatment Study (POTS) demonstrated that combination therapy with medication and cognitive behavioral therapy (CBT) is most effective for moderate to severe OCD. Selective serotonin reuptake inhibitors (SSRIs) are the first-line class of medications used to treat OCD in children and adolescents based on data from double-blind, placebo-controlled trials. All SSRIs seem to be equally effective, although only sertraline (for ages six years and older), fluoxetine (for ages seven years and older), fluvoxamine (for ages eight years and older), and paroxetine (for adults only) have Food and Drug Administration (FDA) approval for the treatment of OCD. Additionally, the tricyclic antidepressant (TCA) clomipramine is FDA approved for the treatment of OCD in children and adolescents ages 10 years and older; however, SSRIs are preferred as the first-line option due to their favorable side effect and toxicity profile. Clinical features associated with poorer response to medication treatment include comorbid tics, poor insight, parental accommodation, and comorbid autism spectrum disorder. Selective serotonin reuptake inhibitors should be used at a therapeutic dose for at least eight and often up to 12 weeks to determine whether the patient experiences a response. It is generally advised to continue the SSRI for at least one year after remission is achieved to prevent symptomatic re-emergence; however, many patients will require longer-term treatment with medications. Adjunctive medications that can be considered if adequate improvement is not achieved with monotherapy include combining an SSRI with clomipramine or second-generation antipsychotic such as risperidone or aripiprazole.

PSYCHOSOCIAL TREATMENT

Cognitive behavioral therapy with a focus on exposure and response prevention (ERP) is the gold standard psychotherapy treatment for OCD. Exposure and response prevention consists of gradual exposure to feared stimuli and prevention of compulsive behaviors. In most ERP protocols for children and adolescents, the treatment begins with psychoeducation about OCD, followed by identifying and cataloging obsessions and compulsions to determine how OCD is affecting the child's life. This process is important for building motivation to engage in treatment. The child is then introduced to anxiety management techniques to "boss back" OCD before engaging in ERP sessions. Exposure includes exposing the child to the thoughts, images, objects, and situations that trigger anxiety. In response prevention, the child endures the anxiety without engaging in the compulsion. As ERP is repeated, the fear and anxiety gradually diminish. Treatment modifications for younger children include greater parental involvement, incorporating games or play into the exposures, and developing a story or narrative to explain and externalize OCD.

Family support groups are recommended for the family members of people with OCD and can favorably contribute to symptom improvement in OCD-affected individuals. The International OCD Foundation has published a website with resources for parents of children and adolescents with OCD (https://kids.iocdf.org/for-parents/).

- Obsessive-compulsive disorder is a relatively common condition, but because youth may hide their symptoms, it often goes underrecognized and untreated.
- Obsessions are ego-dystonic, repetitive, intrusive thoughts, while compulsions consist of difficult-to-control urges to perform certain behaviors or mental acts.
- The CY-BOCS is the gold standard rating scale for assessing and tracking symptom severity.
- The primary treatment for OCD is CBT with ERP therapy combined with an SSRI.

Further Reading

Burchi E, Pallanti S. Diagnostic issues in early-onset obsessive-compulsive disorder and their treatment implications. *Curr Neuropharmacol* 2019;17(8):672–680.

Eisen JL, Mancebo MA, Pinto A, et al. Impact of obsessive-compulsive disorder on quality of life. *Compr Psychiatry* 2006;47(4):270–275.

Grant JE. Obsessive-compulsive disorder. *N Engl J Med* 2014;371(7):646–653.

Hirschtritt ME, Bloch MH, Mathews CA. Obsessive-compulsive disorder: Advances in diagnosis and treatment. *JAMA* 2017;317(13):1358–1367.

Lipton MG, Brewin CR, Linke S, et al. Distinguishing features of intrusive images in obsessive-compulsive disorder. *J Anxiety Disord* 2010;24:816–822.

Nazeer A, Latif F, Mondal A, et al. Obsessive-compulsive disorder in children and adolescents: Epidemiology, diagnosis, and management. *Transl Pediatr* 2020;9:S76–S93.

Ruscio AM, Stein DJ, Chiu WT, et al. The epidemiology of obsessive-compulsive disorder in the National Comorbidity Survey Replication. *Mol Psychiatry* 2010;15:53–63.

Skoog G, Skoog I. A 40-year follow-up of patients with obsessive-compulsive disorder. *Arch Gen Psychiatry* 1999;56:121–127.

Thomsen PH. Obsessions: The impact and treatment of obsessive-compulsive disorder in children and adolescents. *J Psychopharmacol* 2000;14(2):S31–S37.

18 A girl without stranger danger

Lauren N. Deaver

A five-year-old girl and her adoptive mother present for a psychiatric evaluation for inappropriate social behaviors. The patient was adopted one year ago from an international orphanage. At first, she appeared to bond well with her new parents, turning to them for comfort when distressed. However, her parents noticed she is friendly and talkative with all adults, regardless of familiarity. Her parents are concerned she might walk away with a stranger.

The patient was reportedly removed from her biological parents' custody around the age of one year for severe neglect and lived in an orphanage until her adoption occurred. When she arrived in the United States, she was in good physical health without signs of malnutrition.

Upon meeting the psychiatrist, the patient approaches him for a hug. She requests that the psychiatrist take her to the front desk to choose a sticker. She leaves the exam room and does not check back with her adoptive parents before doing so.

What Do You Do Now?

This is a case of disinhibited social engagement disorder (DSED), which is categorized as a Trauma- and Stressor-Related Disorder in the *Diagnostic and Statistical Manual of Mental Disorders*, Fifth Edition (DSM-5). Children with DSED exhibit disinhibited social behaviors, most notably a willingness to approach, interact with, and even leave with unfamiliar adults. To meet criteria for DSED, the child must have experienced extreme neglect or abuse, such as being reared in an institution. Socially indiscriminate behaviors are adaptive in institutional environments, allowing emotionally neglected children to receive short bursts of attunement or affection. However, these same behaviors are highly maladaptive outside of institutions, as they place the child at risk of abduction. Disinhibited social engagement disorder may co-occur with developmental delays, stereotypic behaviors, malnutrition, or other signs of abuse and neglect. After the child is removed from the neglectful environment, the disinhibited social behaviors may persist even after other signs and symptoms of early childhood neglect have resolved. Signs of DSED may also persist after the child has formed secure attachments with his or her caregivers. Disinhibited social engagement disorder significantly impairs a child's ability to interpersonally relate to adults and peers. When symptoms persist into adolescence, they are associated with increased peer conflict. Little is known about the natural history and longitudinal outcomes associated with this disorder in adulthood. In general, children who have experienced extreme neglect are at higher risk of developing psychiatric disorders including major depressive disorder (MDD), bipolar disorder, generalized anxiety disorder (GAD), posttraumatic stress disorder (PTSD), and substance use disorders in adolescence and adulthood.

EPIDEMIOLOGY

Disinhibited social engagement disorder appears to be rare, although its true prevalence is unknown. Only a small number of children who experience extreme neglect or abuse will go on to develop DSED. Disinhibited social engagement disorder is one of two disorders, the other being reactive attachment disorder (RAD), that is the sequelae of extreme neglect or abuse during early childhood. Classically, DSED is described in children who were institutionalized in settings with high child-to-caregiver ratios and where caregivers work in shifts. It also may develop in children who experience extreme deprivation due to parental mental illness, substance abuse, or other factors that impede the parents' ability to provide consistent care. Children with a history of DSED exhibit poorer competencies in adolescence in the areas of family relationships, peer relationships, academic performance, physical health, mental health, substance use, and risk-taking behavior, even when signs of DSED diminished by the age of 12 years. Risk factors for developing DSED include increased time living in institutionalized care and frequent changes in institutional placement. Some studies suggest there may be genetic risk factors for DSED. For example, certain polymorphisms in the serotonin transporter gene (5-HTT) and in the brain-derived neurotrophic factor (BDNF) gene may lead to increased risk for developing indiscriminate social behavior when exposed to extreme neglect.

SIGNS AND SYMPTOMS

A history of extremely insufficient care must be present to meet criteria for the diagnosis of DSED. According to the DSM-5, insufficient care may include extreme social neglect or deprivation leading to a lack of having basic emotional needs including affection, comfort, or stimulation met by caregiving adults; repeated changes of primary caregivers that limit opportunities to form stable attachments; or being raised in unusual settings that limit opportunities to form selective attachments. The hallmark symptom of DSED is exhibiting socially indiscriminate behaviors. The child must exhibit at least two of the following: (1) reduced or no reticence in approaching unfamiliar adults; (2) being verbally or physically overly familiar (that is not consistent with culturally sanctioned or age-appropriate boundaries); (3) diminished or absent checking back with caregiver after venturing away, even in unfamiliar settings; and (4) willingness to leave with an unfamiliar adult with minimal to no hesitation. The child must have a developmental age of at least nine months. In addition, the behaviors must not be solely secondary to impulsivity, such as in attention-deficit/hyperactivity disorder (ADHD), although this is a frequent comorbidity with DSED.

Prior to the publication of the DSM-5, DSED was considered a socially disinhibited subtype of RAD. However, given the differences in phenotype, course, and response to intervention, DSED is now considered a distinct disorder. Compared to children with RAD, children with DSED are typically more sociable and present with brighter affect. They are often intrusive, lack appropriate social boundaries, and can be overly attention seeking. Their social approach tends to be overly familiar and adults may perceive their "friendliness" as superficial and uncomfortable.

ASSESSMENT

There is no single diagnostic test or screening tool for DSED. If DSED is suspected, the clinician should ascertain whether there is a history of severe neglect, foster care, adoption, or institutional rearing. Caregivers should be asked about how the child behaves around unfamiliar adults, and child-caregiver interactions should be observed during the clinic visit. The clinician should ask about and observe for the presence of attachment behaviors including turning preferentially to the caregiver for comfort, showing stranger wariness, and protesting when separation from familiar caregivers occurs. A structured observation paradigm that includes elements of separation from and reunion with the caregiver, as well as interactions with a stranger, may be helpful. Children with secure attachments exhibit a clear preference for the attachment figure and the separation should be mildly stressful. In older children, the clinician should also inquire about socially indiscriminate behaviors with same-age peers. Older children with DSED may have an overly broad or shallow definition of friendship and may claim that they have "close" friendships with relatively new acquaintances.

The clinical assessment should also seek to differentiate DSED from ADHD. The nature of the impulsivity can be used to delineate between these two disorders. In DSED, the impulsivity primarily occurs in the context of social interactions, whereas in ADHD the impulsivity is more diffuse. It should be noted that DSED and ADHD may co-occur. The child should also be assessed for other comorbid psychiatric disorders including intellectual disability, language disorders, and PTSD.

When there are concerns for DSED, the child's safety in the current placement should also be assessed. Children with DSED are at high risk for further victimization, in part due to a higher likelihood of exhibiting challenging behaviors that may be difficult for caregivers to manage. If there are concerns for ongoing neglect or abuse, a report must be made to Child Protective Services.

BIOLOGICAL TREATMENT

There are no biological treatments for DSED. Patients should be screened for comorbid psychiatric disorders such as MDD, bipolar disorder, or GAD. If comorbid psychiatric disorders are present, the child may benefit from pharmacologic treatments for these disorders.

Children with DSED should also undergo a comprehensive medical examination and assessment to ensure that they have received age-appropriate medical and dental care, including vaccinations.

PSYCHOSOCIAL TREATMENT

The cornerstone of treatment for DSED is to provide the child with an emotionally available attachment figure. This may include placement in a foster or adoptive home. The impact of appropriate caregiving on the course of DSED is more variable than in RAD. Children who receive appropriate, emotionally available caregiving may have continuing symptoms of DSED, even after forming a secure attachment with a caregiver. In these instances, the child preferentially seeks comfort from a preferred attachment figure but continues to unhesitatingly approach strangers. The initial priority of the therapeutic intervention should include establishing and developing the attachment relationship. There may also be cases in which limiting a child's exposure to strangers for several months may be helpful in reducing or eliminating the socially indiscriminate behaviors. If the symptoms of DSED are accompanied by oppositional or aggressive behaviors, family-based therapies to address oppositionality such as parent-child interaction therapy (for younger children) or multisystemic therapy (for adolescents) may be helpful.

Raising a child with symptoms of DSED can be challenging. Parents may benefit from parent guidance to support the development of parenting skills that allow them to provide a consistent, nurturing environment for their child. The American Academy of Child and Adolescent Psychiatry (AACAP) has published a Facts for Families document on attachment disorders (https://www.aacap.org/AACAP/Families_and_Youth/Facts_for_Families/FFF-Guide/Attachment-Disorders-085.aspx).

KEY POINTS TO REMEMBER

- A history of insufficient care such as extreme neglect, repeated change of caregivers, or being raised in an unusual environment (institution) must be present.
- Disinhibited social engagement disorder is characterized by socially disinhibited behaviors, most notably a willingness to approach, interact with, and even leave with unfamiliar adults.
- Treatment focuses on providing the child with an emotionally available caregiver and working to develop a secure attachment relationship.
- Symptoms of DSED may persist even after a secure attachment has developed.

Further Reading

Guyon-Harris KL, Humphreys KL, Fox NA, et al. Course of disinhibited social engagement disorder from early childhood to early adolescence. *J Am Acad Child Adoles Psychiatry* 2018;57(5):329–335.

Sanuga-Barke EJS, Kennedy M, Kumsta R, et al. Child-to-adult neurodevelopment and mental health trajectories after early life deprivation: The young adult follow-up of the longitudinal English and Romanian adoptees study. *Lancet* 2017;389:1539–1548.

Zeanah CH, Chester T, Boris NW. Practice parameter for the assessment and treatment of children and adolescents with reactive attachment disorder and disinhibited social engagement disorder. *J Am Acad Child Adoles Psychiatry* 2016;55(11):990–1003.

Zeanah CH, Gleason MM. Annual research review: Attachment disorders in early childhood: Clinical presentation, causes, correlates, and treatment. *J Child Psychol Psychiatry* 2015;56:207–222.

19 A boy who could not be comforted

Katherine A. Epstein

A seven-year-old boy is accompanied by his adoptive father to a psychiatric evaluation for severe tantrums. Since arriving in his adoptive home eight months ago, he has had severe tantrums several times per week. During these tantrums, when his parents try to help him calm down, he screams and physically attacks them. When he has a minor injury, like scraping his knee, he responds to his parents' attempts to soothe him by saying, "Stop, you are hurting me!" The patient is not affectionate and often makes statements such as "I don't want to be part of this family."

Until the age of four years, the patient lived with his biological parents, who had severe mental illness and substance use disorders. He was sexually abused, witnessed violence between his parents, and was eventually removed from his parents' custody. He subsequently spent time in two different foster homes where he was physically abused, before finally being adopted by his current parents.

What Do You Do Now?

The patient is suffering from reactive attachment disorder (RAD), one of two disorders, along with disinhibited social engagement disorder (DSED), that is the result of extreme neglect or abuse during early childhood. Both of these disorders are evident before the age of five years and occur when a young child is deprived of the opportunity to form a secure attachment with a reliable caregiver. These disorders are classically observed in children who are institutionalized in settings with high child-to-caregiver ratios and where caregivers work in shifts. However, it can also affect children who experience extreme deprivation due to parental mental illness, substance abuse, or other factors that impede the parents' ability to provide consistent care. Children with RAD demonstrate the absence of social reciprocity toward caregivers, fail to seek or receive comfort, and have difficulty with emotional regulation. Identifying RAD is important because the treatment, providing the child the opportunity to form a secure attachment, is both specific and effective. Additionally, the symptoms of RAD can be very distressing and confusing to adoptive parents.

Data on the long-term outcomes of children with RAD is very limited. However, early childhood neglect is also associated with decreased cognitive ability and attention-deficit/hyperactivity disorder. Children with a history of extreme neglect also have higher rates of major depressive disorder (MDD), bipolar disorder, generalized anxiety disorder (GAD), posttraumatic stress disorder, and substance use disorders in adolescence and adulthood.

EPIDEMIOLOGY

A prerequisite for the diagnosis of RAD is exposure to pathogenic care before the age of five years. Although definitive prevalence studies of RAD are lacking, RAD is thought to be quite rare, even among children who have been exposed to severe abuse or neglect. Most of what we know about RAD comes from the Bucharest Early Intervention Project, a randomized controlled trial of foster care as an intervention for children abandoned at or around the time of birth in Bucharest, Romania. One-hundred and thirty-six children were randomly assigned to either high-quality foster care or to remain in institutional care. The average age at randomization was 22 months. At the time of randomization, 5% of children met criteria for RAD. The children were followed at regular intervals up until the age of 12 years. Among the orphans who were fostered, the degree of RAD symptomatology was comparable to the never-institutionalized group by 30 months of age. Those who remained institutionalized had stable signs of RAD through eight years of age.

Children with lower cognitive abilities are at increased risk for developing symptoms of RAD. Risk factors for persistent RAD include more placement disruptions and increased time living in institutional care. Medical and psychiatric comorbidities that can co-occur with RAD include developmental delays, malnutrition, MDD, and stereotypic movement disorder.

SIGNS AND SYMPTOMS

According to the *Diagnostic and Statistical Manual of Mental Disorders*, Fifth Edition (DSM-5), a prerequisite for the diagnosis of RAD is a history of extremely insufficient care. Insufficient care can include a persistent lack of having basic emotional needs for comfort, stimulation, and affection met by caregiving adults; repeated changes of primary caregivers that limit opportunities to form stable attachments (e.g., frequent changes in foster care); or being raised in an unusual setting that severely limits the opportunity to form selective attachments (e.g., institutions with high child-to-caregiver ratios). Children with RAD exhibit a consistent pattern of inhibited, emotionally withdrawn behavior toward adult caregivers, manifesting as rarely seeking and responding to comfort when distressed. Additionally, the child has persistent social and emotional disturbance characterized by at least two of minimal social and emotional responsiveness to others; limited positive affect; and episodes of unexplained irritability, sadness, or fearfulness that are evident even during nonthreatening interactions with caregivers. To make this diagnosis, a child must be old enough to be developmentally capable of forming a selective attachment (older than nine months) and demonstrate symptoms before the age of five years.

Reactive attachment disorder is considered to be behaviorally distinct from DSED, the other disorder resulting from extreme abuse or neglect before the age of five years, which reflects the current DSM-5 classification. However, in previous editions of the DSM, RAD was divided into two subtypes: the emotionally withdrawn subtype, now known as RAD, and the socially disinhibited subtype, now known as DSED.

ASSESSMENT

The assessment of RAD should include a clinical history that screens for exposure to extremes of insufficient care such as growing up with parents who are unable to care for their children, multiple foster placements, or spending time in an institutional setting. Because RAD is a disorder of selective attachment, it is essential to interview the child's primary caregiver to assess the nature of the attachment relationship. The first five items in the Disturbance of Attachment Interview, a rating scale widely used in RAD and DSED research, can be helpful in assessing the attachment relationship. This rating scale is a semistructured interview that is administered to the child's primary caregiver. The first five items, relevant to RAD, ask if the patient (1) differentiates among adults; (2) seeks comfort preferentially from a preferred caregiver; (3) responds to caregivers when hurt, frightened, or distressed; (4) responds reciprocally with familiar caregivers; and (5) regulates emotions well with ample positive and developmentally expected levels of irritability and/or sadness. Direct observation of the parent-child relationship and interactions can also aid in making the diagnosis. The clinician should observe the parent's capacity for empathy, level of responsiveness, and emotional reactions to the child. The child's responsiveness to the parent and bids for attention or comfort should also be observed. Pertinent mental status examination observations may include appearing withdrawn, passive, or disinterested in people.

The initial assessment should also screen for ongoing abuse or neglect, including information about interactions with parents/caregivers as well as other adults in the home environment. If the diagnosis of RAD is suspected, the child should undergo a complete physical examination and medical evaluation for signs and symptoms of malnutrition, abuse, or neglect.

The differential diagnosis for RAD includes other disorders that can diminish positive affect and/or disrupt social relationships. Like RAD, autism spectrum disorder (ASD) can blunt the expression of positive emotions and impair social reciprocity. However, unlike RAD, ASD is not usually associated with a history of neglect. Moreover, the diagnostic criteria for RAD do not include restricted, repetitive patterns of behavior, which is a core feature of ASD. Disorders that are associated with emotion dysregulation, including mood disorders, should also be included on the differential diagnosis for RAD. However, young children with MDD should still be capable of forming selective attachments and can be distinguished from children with RAD in this way.

BIOLOGICAL TREATMENT

There are no biological treatments that specifically target RAD symptoms, although screening for and treating comorbid psychiatric disorders, such as MDD, bipolar disorder, or GAD, are indicated.

A child with RAD should undergo a medical examination and comprehensive assessment to ensure that they have received age-appropriate medical and dental care, including vaccinations.

PSYCHOSOCIAL TREATMENT

The single effective treatment for RAD is facilitating placement of the child in an environment where they have the opportunity to form a selective attachment to a caregiver. If there is concern for ongoing child abuse or neglect, the clinician is mandated to report this concern to Child Protective Services. Child Protective Services would then determine whether the report is substantiated, and if so, determine which interventions are needed, ranging from voluntarily accepted supports in the home, such as family therapy or parent training, to taking emergency custody of the child.

Although the symptoms of RAD may dissipate, children who have a history of institutionalization or extreme neglect or abuse remain at elevated risk for psychiatric disorders across the lifespan. The intervention of giving children the opportunity to form a selective attachment decreases, but does not eliminate, the risk of these negative outcomes.

Children with RAD may benefit from individual psychotherapy to increase their ability to identify and regulate emotions, as well as to form secure relationships. Play therapy, which allows for the free expression of thoughts and emotions through play within a safe relationship, may be one such approach, particularly for younger children.

Raising a child with symptoms of RAD can be extremely challenging. Parents may benefit from parent guidance to support the development of parenting skills that allow them to provide a consistent, nurturing environment for the child. The American Academy of Child and Adolescent Psychiatry (AACAP) has published a Facts for Families document on attachment disorders (https://www.aacap.org/AACAP/Families_and_Youth/Facts_for_Families/FFF-Guide/Attachment-Disorders-085.aspx).

KEY POINTS TO REMEMBER

- Reactive attachment disorder is one of two disorders that can result when a child is deprived of the opportunity to form a selective attachment with a caregiver.
- Reactive attachment disorder is rare, occurring in about 5% of institutionalized children.
- Children with RAD demonstrate the absence of social reciprocity toward caregivers, fail to seek or receive comfort, and have disturbances in emotional regulation.
- Reactive attachment disorder can be effectively treated by giving a child the opportunity to form a selective attachment. Symptoms may completely resolve if this occurs.
- The symptoms of RAD are much more amenable to intervention than the symptoms of DSED.
- Even after symptoms of RAD resolve, patients with a history of extreme abuse or neglect remain at risk for developing other psychiatric disorders later in life.

Further Reading

Gleason MM, Fox NA, Drury S, et al. Validity of evidence-derived criteria for reactive attachment disorder: Indiscriminately social/disinhibited and emotionally withdrawn/inhibited types. *J Am Acad Child Adolesc Psychiatry* 2011;50:216–231. e213.

Humphreys KL, Gleason MM, Drury SS, et al. Effects of institutional rearing and foster care on psychopathology at age 12 years in Romania: Follow-up of an open, randomised controlled trial. *Lancet Psychiatry* 2015;2:625–634.

Humphreys KL, Nelson CA, Fox NA, et al. Signs of reactive attachment disorder and disinhibited social engagement disorder at age 12 years: Effects of institutional care history and high-quality foster care. *Dev Psychopathol* 2017;29:675–684.

Smyke AT, Dumitrescu A, Zeanah CH. Attachment disturbances in young children. I: The continuum of caretaking casualty. *J Am Acad Child Adolesc Psychiatry* 2002;41:972–982.

Smyke AT, Zeanah CH, Gleason MM, et al. A randomized controlled trial comparing foster care and institutional care for children with signs of reactive attachment disorder. *Am J Psychiatry* 2012;169:508–514.

Zeanah CH, Gleason MM. Annual research review: Attachment disorders in early childhood—Clinical presentation, causes, correlates, and treatment. *J Child Psychol Psychiatry* 2015;56:207–222.

20 Sad mood and changes in behavior after exposure to a traumatic reminder

Joshua R. Smith

An 11-year-old girl presents to the psychiatry clinic with her adoptive parents. She was in foster care, where she was physically abused by her foster brother, until the age of seven years. There was also concern for sexual abuse. Since her adoption four years ago, the patient has had poor self-esteem and experiences recurrent nightmares.

Recently, her parents have been preparing her to transition from homeschool to middle school, attending for a few hours each week. One week ago, she encountered her foster brother in the school hallway. She began to hyperventilate and cry, and attempted to cut her forearm with a pen. Since then, she has refused to return to school. Her adoptive parents feel guilty about this, as they didn't think she would see her foster brother at school.

You ask about the episode of self-injury with the pen. She explains that when she was being abused by her foster brother, she would try to cut herself with blunt objects to "get rid" of the pain he caused her.

What Do You Do Now?

The patient is likely suffering from an acute exacerbation of chronic posttraumatic stress disorder (PTSD). The accurate identification and treatment of PTSD in children and adolescents is critical, given the long-term risks of untreated PTSD including suicide attempts, substance use, major depressive disorder (MDD), and ongoing functional impairments.

EPIDEMIOLOGY

Traumatic experiences are common in childhood and adolescence. One in four individuals experiences a traumatic event before reaching adulthood. The specific content of these traumatic events is wide ranging and includes but is not limited to domestic or community violence, natural disasters, car accidents, medical trauma, or the death of a loved one. After a traumatic event, most children will either experience time-limited traumatic response symptoms or remain asymptomatic. However, some children develop impairing traumatic response symptoms that are chronic. Overall, 3% to 6% of children who experience any trauma and 40% of children who experience sexual trauma will develop symptoms meeting the diagnostic criteria for PTSD. Notably, many other children experience trauma response symptoms that do not fully meet criteria for PTSD but result in functional impairments that are equivalent to those associated with PTSD.

Risk factors for the development of PTSD include female gender, previous and repeated traumatic exposure, poverty, parental mental illness or substance abuse, lower academic achievement, isolation, minority status, and pre-existing psychiatric disorders. Risk factors for developing PTSD after experiencing a disaster-related trauma include increased exposure to disaster-related events in the media, delayed evacuation from the disaster zone, or having felt that a family member's life was in danger. Protective factors include parental support, lower levels of parental PTSD, self-efficacy and problem-solving skills, stable relationships, community supports, positive relationships with caregivers, higher socioeconomic status, religious affiliation, and older age at the time of traumatic exposure.

Long-term clinical outcomes of children and adolescents with PTSD are variable. Chronic PTSD, defined as persistent or episodic symptomatology and functional impairment, is associated with poorer outcomes. Additionally, psychiatric comorbidity with MDD, substance use disorders, anxiety disorders, and attention-deficit/hyperactivity disorder (ADHD) is common.

SIGNS AND SYMPTOMS

The *Diagnostic and Statistical Manual for Mental Disorders*, Fifth Edition (DSM-5), classifies PTSD as a trauma- and stressor-related disorder. According to the DSM-5, to meet criteria for PTSD, the individual must have had exposure to a traumatic event. Trauma is defined in the DSM-5 as actual or threatened death, serious injury, or violence. The exposure can occur by directly experiencing the event, witnessing (in person) the event as it occurred to others, learning that the traumatic event occurred to a close friend or family member, or experiencing repeated or extreme exposure to aversive details of the traumatic event. Beyond establishing a history of exposure to trauma, the diagnostic criteria are different for persons six years and younger and seven years and older. This distinction is present to ensure that the diagnostic criteria for PTSD are developmentally appropriate.

For children and adolescents older than seven years, exposure to a traumatic event must be accompanied by one month or more of intrusion symptoms, avoidance of stimuli associated with the traumatic event, negative alterations in cognitions and mood, and marked alterations in arousal and reactivity associated with the traumatic event. Intrusion symptoms may present as recurrent, involuntary, and intrusive distressing memories of the event; recurrent distressing dreams about the traumatic event; flashbacks in which the individual feels or acts as if the traumatic event were recurring; or prolonged psychological/physiological distress when exposed to internal or external cues that symbolize the traumatic event. Compared to adults, intrusion symptoms in children older than six years may manifest as repetitive play in which themes from or aspects of the trauma are expressed. Trauma-specific reenactment may also occur in play. Children are often unaware of the connection between their repetitive play and the trauma. Finally, children may experience frightening dreams without recognizable content. Avoidance behaviors include persistent efforts to avoid distressing recollections or reminders (e.g., people, places, activities, situations) of the traumatic event. Mood or cognitive changes may include amnesia, persistent negative beliefs about oneself, self-blame, anhedonia, feelings of detachment from others, and an inability to experience positive emotions. Symptoms of changes in arousal include irritability, self-destructive behavior, hypervigilance, exaggerated startle response, problems with concentration, or sleep disturbance. If symptoms resolve within one month, the diagnosis of acute stress disorder is made rather than PTSD.

The DSM-5 diagnostic criteria for PTSD in children six years and younger include a greater emphasis on witnessing or learning that traumatic events occurred to a caregiver, as a child's loss of parent/caregiver stability may be experienced as a trauma. Patients in this age range continue to require the presence of at least one symptom from each of the four symptom clusters described previously for at least one month to meet the diagnostic criteria. However, specific descriptions of criteria include developmental considerations. Intrusive thoughts may be experienced as play reenactment and distressing dreams may or may not include traumatic content. Negative cognitive alterations are also described as constriction in play and developmental regression. Posttraumatic stress disorder can also present with new-onset symptoms of oppositionality or separation anxiety in both children and adolescents.

Finally, specifiers for the diagnosis of PTSD are applicable to all age ranges. These include dissociative symptoms with either depersonalization (feeling detached from one's mental processes or body) or derealization (experiences of unreality of one's surroundings) and PTSD with delayed expression. The latter occurs if full diagnostic criteria are not met until at least six months after the traumatic event occurred.

ASSESSMENT

Taking a developmental approach is vital in the diagnostic assessment of pediatric PTSD. Preschool, preadolescent, and adolescent youth will have significant variability in their ability to describe traumatic events and complex emotional states. Similarly, it has been reported that nearly 88% of PTSD symptomatology is not observable from a clinical examination of young children, further complicating the assessment.

Providing psychoeducation to the child and/or caregiver about the complexity of trauma-related symptomatology reduces the risk of over- or underreporting of symptoms. This is particularly true in cases of parents who have not experienced trauma and are reporting symptoms on behalf of their children. Additionally, inclusion of the caregiver in the evaluation improves diagnostic accuracy and should be done whenever possible. After an initial evaluation, collateral information from community supports such as teachers or coaches may also be useful to learn about the child's behavior and functioning in a variety of settings.

When inquiring about symptoms and their relation to a traumatic event, it is important to recognize that a common feature of PTSD is the inability to recall specific events about the trauma. Thus, the interviewer should tailor questions to make them more specific to the patient's circumstances rather than asking broad, open-ended questions. For example, the interviewer could ask, "When you see your foster brother at school, do you have strong feelings or get upset?" Since avoidance is a core symptom of PTSD, open-ended lines of questioning may result in underreporting of symptoms.

Given the diagnostic challenges in the assessment of younger children, validated screening measures may be of assistance. There are two screening instruments that are specifically designed for patients as young as three years. The Traumatic Experiences Screening Instrument is a 15- to 24-item clinician-administered (for ages three to 17 years) or child self-report (for ages 11 to 17 years) rating scale to measure exposure to interpersonal, noninterpersonal, or traumatic victimization. The Trauma Symptom Checklist for Young Children (TSCYC) and Children (TSCC) is validated for patients three to 17 years of age. The TSCYC utilizes parent report, while the TSCC relies on self-report from the child. Although formal neuropsychological testing is not required to diagnose PTSD, it can be helpful in determining cognitive pathology and specific impairments.

Multiple psychiatric conditions may present with symptoms similar to those seen in PTSD. On mental status examination, children with PTSD can present with variable levels of psychomotor activity, from slowed to hyperactive. Cognitive symptoms, sleep disturbances, social withdrawal, and self-injury are also common. Thus, children may be inaccurately diagnosed with ADHD, bipolar disorder, MDD, or oppositional defiant disorder. There is also overlap with symptoms of panic disorder, obsessive-compulsive disorder (OCD), generalized anxiety disorder (GAD), and specific phobia based on fear responses, cognitive alterations, and physiological hyperarousal to traumatic reminders. Posttraumatic stress disorder may also be misdiagnosed as a primary substance use disorder when drugs or alcohol are used for emotional numbing or avoidance. Psychotic disorders may also be on the differential diagnosis, since children who have experienced trauma may experience perceptual disturbances related to the trauma and can present as severely agitated. Thus, careful evaluation for a history of exposure to trauma is key in distinguishing PTSD from other psychiatric conditions.

Multiple medical conditions including asthma, hyperthyroidism, substance intoxication, seizure disorder, migraines, and catecholamine- or serotonin-secreting tumors may also present similarly to PTSD. Further complicating the clinical picture, PTSD often presents with somatic symptoms including headaches and abdominal pain. A thorough medical examination of a child who has been exposed to trauma should be part of the diagnostic workup. Similarly, a mental health evaluation of children presenting to pediatrics with somatic complaints is warranted.

LEVEL OF CARE

Children with PTSD often present with self-injury and are more likely to attempt suicide when compared to their nontraumatized peers. The etiology and rationale of self-injury or suicidal ideation, access to emergency resources, firearm safety, caregiver involvement, and access to lethal means such as medication stockpiles should be considered when determining the most appropriate level of care. If a patient has limited social supports, is actively engaging in self-harm, minimally participates in the interview or safety planning, or has ego-syntonic suicidal ideation with a plan and access to means, an inpatient level of care would likely be warranted. Alternatively, if the patient is experiencing ego-dystonic suicidal ideation, is participating actively in treatment, and has support systems in place that he or she can access, lower levels of care such as a partial hospital program or outpatient care may be considered.

PREVENTION

On average, PTSD symptoms develop one month after the exposure to a traumatic event. How this delay between exposure to the traumatic event and symptom onset can best be used to decrease the risk of developing PTSD is an active area of research. Helping both the child and caregiver to build resilience through enhancing self-care skills, emotional intelligence, and mindfulness-based practices may be of benefit.

Community involvement and screening after a societal-level traumatic event is important for early identification. Screening ideally occurs within one month of the traumatic event. Interventions such as the Cognitive Behavioral Intervention for Trauma in Schools (CBITS) can provide early treatment for children with PTSD symptoms. This is done to provide education on the impact of trauma as it relates to classroom behavior. In diverse community samples exposed to trauma, CBITS has proven superior to a waitlist control condition in the reduction of PTSD and depressive symptomatology.

BIOLOGICAL TREATMENT

Two selective serotonin reuptake inhibitors (SSRIs), paroxetine and sertraline, are Food and Drug Administration (FDA) approved for the treatment of PTSD in adults. However, the evidence supporting their use in pediatric patients is mixed. Two open-label studies of citalopram showed that child and adolescent patients experienced a reduction of PTSD symptoms. However, a large randomized controlled trial of sertraline found that sertraline was not superior to placebo. Another controlled study comparing fluoxetine, imipramine, and placebo in treating children with acute stress disorder found that neither medication was superior to placebo. Thus, it is generally preferable to begin with psychotherapeutic interventions before initiating an SSRI. There is also concern that SSRIs may be overly activating in some patients and may result in worsened symptomatology. However, children with comorbid conditions that are responsive to medications including MDD, OCD, and GAD should receive SSRIs earlier in the treatment course.

Other classes of medications that require further research but may be considered include alpha$_1$ adrenergic antagonists, alpha$_2$ adrenergic agonists, and beta-blockers. Case studies suggest that prazosin, an alpha$_1$ adrenergic antagonist, may be safe and effective for pediatric PTSD. Open-label studies have found that the alpha$_2$ adrenergic agonists clonidine and guanfacine may be helpful in decreasing hyperarousal and re-experiencing symptoms. Finally, propranolol, a beta-blocker, may help decrease the physical symptoms associated with hyperarousal.

PSYCHOSOCIAL TREATMENT

Psychosocial interventions are the gold standard treatment for PTSD. Multiple different modalities of psychotherapy have been found to be effective. Regardless of modality, critical components of treatment include a trauma-focused approach that specifically addresses the child's traumatic experiences, involving the parent/caregiver as an important agent of change, and a focus on symptom reduction to improve functioning and resilience and allow for resumption of normal development. Evidence suggests that incorporating these approaches results in greater symptom reduction across the developmental spectrum.

Trauma-focused cognitive behavioral therapy (TF-CBT) has the greatest empirical support for pediatric PTSD. Components of this treatment can be described with the acronym PRACTICE: Psychoeducation and Parenting skills, Relaxation skills, Affective modulation skills, Cognitive coping and processing, Trauma narrative, In vivo mastery of trauma reminders, Conjoint child-parent sessions, and Enhancing future safety and development. The American Academy of Child and Adolescent Psychiatry (AACAP) has published a Facts for Families article that may be used to help educate families about PTSD and increase awareness of symptoms and functional impairments (https://www.aacap.org/AACAP/Families_ and_Youth/Facts_for_Families/FFF-Guide/Posttraumatic-Stress-Disorder-PTSD-070.aspx).

Psychodynamic psychotherapy for trauma has also been shown to be an effective means of treatment. This modality focuses on personality coherence, healthy development, and symptom reduction. In younger children, the focus is on the parent-child relationship rather than the individual. Child-parent psychotherapy is a treatment model for young children who have experienced domestic violence, which combines components of attachment theory and TF-CBT. Components include modeling appropriate protective behavior, assisting the parent in accurately interpreting the child's actions and emotions, and developing a joint parent-child narrative about the trauma.

· Children who experience traumatic events but do not meet full criteria for PTSD often suffer from similar functional limitations.
· A developmental perspective is vital in assessing for PTSD in children and adolescents.
· Regardless of the psychotherapeutic modality, key features of effective treatment include addressing the trauma, involving the parents/caregivers as agents of change, and focusing on both symptoms and functionality.
· No biologic treatments are FDA approved for pediatric PTSD, but using medications to treat psychiatric comorbidities likely improves clinical outcomes.
· A careful risk assessment should occur during each clinical encounter given elevated risks of self-injury and suicide attempts.

Further Reading

Cohen JA, Bukstein O, Walter H, et al. Practice parameter for the assessment and treatment of children and adolescents with posttraumatic stress disorder. *J Am Acad Child Adolesc Psychiatry* 2010;49(4):17.

Cohen J, Mannarino A, Deblinger E. *Treating Trauma and Traumatic Grief in Children and Adolescents.* New York: Guilford Press, 2006.

Connor DF, Ford JD, Arnsten AFT, et al. An update on posttraumatic stress disorder in children and adolescents. *Clin Pediatr (Phila)* 2015;54(6):517–528.

Ortiz R. Building resilience against the sequelae of adverse childhood experiences: Rise up, change your life, and reform health care. *Am J Lifestyle Med* 2019;13(5):470–479.

Stein BD, Jaycox LH, Kataoka SH, et al. A mental health intervention for schoolchildren exposed to violence: A randomized controlled trial. *JAMA* 2003;290(5):603.

21 A child whose parent insists on recurrent medical admissions

Lauren N. Deaver

A four-year-old boy is hospitalized for the fifth time in the past year for the evaluation of seizures. His mother reports multiple seizures per day unresponsive to antiepileptic medications. She also reports a speech delay and gait impairment. Medical record review reveals the patient has been evaluated by multiple pediatric neurologists from several institutions. Prior records document a normal neurological examination, electroencephalogram (EEG), and neuroimaging studies. His mother often requests a second opinion or fails to follow up with a provider after learning of normal results. There is no previous documentation of developmental delay. Hospital staff have never observed seizure-like episodes previously, despite his mother's reports of frequent seizures. During this admission, the patient demonstrates a normal speech pattern and gait when his mother is not present. A routine EEG is normal. There are no seizure events on video-EEG. When the medical team recommends a trial of weaning the patient's antiepileptic medications, his mother demands that he be discharged immediately.

What Do You Do Now?

This is a case of factious disorder imposed on another (FDIA), previously known as Munchausen syndrome by proxy, characterized by the deceptive falsification of illness in another person in the absence of obvious external rewards. In the pediatric setting, it is most often a caregiver who falsifies illness in a child. The caregiver is the one who receives the diagnosis of FDIA and the child is a victim of medical child abuse (MCA). Children who are victims of FDIA are at risk of significant harm. Mortality estimates range from 6% to 9%. There is also a high risk of morbidity and iatrogenesis related to unnecessary diagnostic and therapeutic procedures, for example, the unnecessary placement of a gastric tube for feeding or unnecessary antiepileptic medications. Long-term morbidity may include permanent disfigurement, developmental delay, malnutrition, and the development of psychiatric disorders including anxiety disorders, major depressive disorder, or posttraumatic stress disorder secondary to either the inducement of illness or the medical interventions performed. Victims of FDIA are also at higher risk of developing factitious disorder imposed on self, developing personality disorders, or becoming adult perpetrators of MCA in adulthood.

EPIDEMIOLOGY

The true prevalence of FDIA is unknown. In children under the age of 16 years, the incidence of victimization is estimated to range from 0.5 to 2.0 cases per 100,000. It is suspected that many cases go unrecognized. The perpetrator is most often the biological mother, although other caregivers including fathers, adoptive parents, or other relatives have been reported. Parents may also collude with one another to falsify an illness. Other caregiver risk factors include thriving on attention from physicians, working in a health care profession, and a personal history of a somatic symptom disorder. Boys and girls are equally likely to be victims. Victims are most commonly infants and toddlers (median age at diagnosis: 14 months to 2.7 years), but older children and adolescents may also be affected. The average time from the onset of MCA to diagnosis is estimated to be 15 to 22 months but can take years or never be identified at all. Typically, only one child is targeted at a time, but siblings are also at increased risk for victimization.

SIGNS AND SYMPTOMS

According to the *Diagnostic and Statistical Manual of Mental Disorders*, Fifth Edition (DSM-5), FDIA is characterized by an individual deceptively falsifying illness in another person. The individual presents the victim to others as ill, impaired, or injured. Falsification of illness may include fabricating or exaggerating signs or symptoms, simulating illness (e.g., adding blood to a urine sample), or inducing true illness in the victim (e.g., poisoning or suffocation). The deception occurs in the absence of obvious external rewards such as financial gain or avoiding legal consequences. Fully understanding the intent or motivation of the caregiver is not necessary to make the diagnosis. The perpetrator of MCA, not the child, receives the diagnosis of FDIA.

A wide range of illnesses may be fabricated and the reported symptoms can often be difficult to verify. Common illnesses that are fabricated include apnea, feeding intolerance or food allergies, seizures, chronic vomiting, or diarrhea. There are several warning signs that raise concern for possible FDIA. Aspects of a patient's history may include atypical presentations, multiple medical illnesses, seeking care from multiple institutions or providers, resisting reassurance that the child is healthy, or multiple hospitalizations and surgeries. The medical history may be vague and include inconsistent details. Tests and observations may be normal and inconsistent with the caregiver's report of symptoms. The child's illness may not respond as would be expected to treatment. If the caregiver is absent, the signs and/or reported symptoms may improve or disappear. However, children may also be coached to misrepresent themselves as ill and may even be convinced that they are ill. The caregiver may request further investigations, procedures, or second opinions. They may show little concern when invasive procedures are recommended or advocate for more invasive procedures. Caregivers with FDIA often seek the approval of providers and may have extensive medical knowledge.

ASSESSMENT

Factitious disorder imposed on another is an extremely challenging diagnosis to make, in part due to the wide range of possible falsified signs and symptoms. A very broad range of medical presentations has been described, including virtually every organ system. The reported illness may also affect multiple organ systems and the child may be under the care of multiple specialists. Also, medical providers often do not think to include FDIA on the differential diagnosis, as the generally most effective clinical approach is to trust caregivers to provide truthful and accurate information to the best of their ability. Furthermore, up to 30% of children who are victimized may have a true underlying medical condition that complicates the identification of FDIA. The first step to making the diagnosis is including FDIA in the differential diagnosis when there are warning signs that raise clinician concern. When considering a diagnosis of FDIA, a multidisciplinary team including the primary care physician, subspecialists, nursing staff, a social worker, and the hospital's child protection team should be involved in the assessment.

No single test can conclusively establish the diagnosis of FDIA. The assessment should include a detailed review of reported signs and symptoms as well as objective findings from observations, tests, and interventions in the patient's medical record. The medical record review should seek to determine whether the reported history of illness is credible and whether the child is receiving unnecessary or potentially harmful care. Creating a timeline, table, or another organized recording tool is recommended. The patient's primary care doctor and any subspecialists involved should be contacted as part of the review. Since many physicians may be reluctant to document unconfirmed MCA in the medical record, it is important to contact the physician directly to discuss whether this is of concern. All the physicians involved in the child's care should discuss the case together to come to a consensus regarding ongoing management. It may also be helpful to consult with a pediatrician with specialist training in child abuse when making and disclosing the diagnosis.

The child may require hospital admission for an observation period of their symptoms and of the caregiver-child interactions. The team should set clear goals for the admission. Documentation should explicitly note what is observed versus reported by the caregiver. Caregivers should not be permitted to administer medications or feeds or use medical devices without close supervision by hospital staff. In some cases, covert video surveillance has been utilized. This is a complex and controversial approach that has important ethical, legal, and logistical considerations. If this approach is being considered, the provider should determine whether their institution has written protocols for covert video surveillance, and close coordination among multiple teams including the primary team, consulting teams, ethics team, and child protection team would be required. An alternative approach to covert video surveillance is separating the child from the suspected offending caregiver (discussed later).

The child should be interviewed separately from the caregiver and the interview should focus on gathering information on the child's recollection of symptom onset and evolution, as well as a detailed social history. It may also be necessary to separate the child from the caregiver for a more extended period of time during the assessment to determine whether the child's presentation changes when the caregiver is not present. Child Protective Services would need to be involved to legally establish and maintain the separation. The child would need to be monitored for improvement in symptoms in the absence of the caregiver. In addition, treatments believed to be unnecessary should be discontinued and the child monitored to assess how the symptoms respond to discontinuing these treatments.

BIOLOGICAL TREATMENT

There are no specific biological treatments for FDIA. For the child, treatment focuses on limiting unnecessary or harmful medical care. Unnecessary interventions and treatments must be identified and discontinued, starting with the most invasive or dangerous ones. For example, if the child has had a gastric tube placed but tolerates oral intake, removing the gastric tube should be prioritized. Unnecessary medications should also be tapered or discontinued, as medically appropriate.

PSYCHOSOCIAL TREATMENT

Ensuring the safety of the child is the most important aspect of treatment. Since health care providers are mandated reporters, a report to Child

Protective Services must be made. Child Protective Services may recommend an out-of-home placement and/or may take legal custody of the child. Providers should be aware that after a report to Child Protective Services has been made, the caregiver's behavior may escalate in an attempt to prove that the child has an illness. Furthermore, if the child is removed from the home, the caregiver may begin to target other children. Initiating individual psychotherapy is critical for addressing the psychological harm associated with the victimization associated with FDIA. Children may have distorted views of their own health and lack trust in their caregivers as well as the medical system.

It is equally important for the caregiver to engage in psychologic treatment, although adherence and follow-up are often limited. Without intervention, there is significant risk that the caregiver will continue to falsify illness in other people. Approximately 40% of children experience ongoing victimization after the initial diagnosis of FDIA is made. Successful treatment is evidenced by the caregiver acknowledging and describing the abuse, experiencing an appropriate emotional reaction to the harm caused, developing coping strategies to fulfill their emotional needs without harming the child, and demonstrating these skills over time under close supervision.

KEY POINTS TO REMEMBER

- Factious disorder imposed on another is characterized by a caregiver purposefully fabricating illness in a vulnerable person.
- The child is a victim of MCA.
- While uncommon, this disorder is potentially lethal, with mortality estimates of 6% to 9%.
- Assessment requires a multidisciplinary team, review of the medical record, and a possible period of in-hospital observation and/or separation from the caregiver.
- Treatment of the child focuses on ensuring safety, discontinuing unnecessary medical care, and providing psychotherapy.

Further Reading

Bools CN, Neale BA, Meadow SR. Follow up of victims of fabricated illness (Munchausen syndrome by proxy). *Arch Dis Child* 1993;69(6):625–630.

Hall DE, Eubanks L, Meyyazhagan LS, et al. Evaluation of covert video surveillance in the diagnosis of Munchausen syndrome by proxy: Lessons from 41 cases. *Pediatrics* 2000;105(6):1305–1312.

Jenny C, Metz JB. Medical child abuse and medical neglect. *Pediatr Rev* 2020;41(2):49–60.

McClure RJ, Davis PM, Meadow SR, et al. Epidemiology of Munchausen syndrome by proxy, non-accidental poisoning, and non-accidental suffocation. *Arch Dis Child* 1996;75(1):57–61.

22 Decreased food intake after a choking incident

Kathryn S. Czepiel

Lucas is an 11-year-old boy brought to the emergency department for abdominal pain. Lucas describes the pain as crampy, almost constant, and worse after eating. He has nausea and vomiting, but no diarrhea or bloody stools. Lucas has always been a picky eater. This worsened four months ago after Lucas choked on a piece of steak.

A week after choking, Lucas was eating less solid food, like pudding, ice cream, and nutritional shakes. He has a decreased appetite and lost 15 pound over the past two months. There is a family history of anxiety disorders.

On physical examination, Lucas is anxious appearing, and small for his age with diffuse muscle wasting. He has orthostatic hypotension and tachycardia. He has a scaphoid abdomen with diminished bowel sounds.

Lucas's dad explains that this is their fourth trip to an emergency department in the past week. They are frustrated by the lack of diagnosis, as prior imaging and laboratory studies have been normal.

What Do You Do Now?

It will be important to first acquire all previous records from the outside hospitals to exclude the possibility of a diagnosable medical condition. The differential diagnosis for abdominal pain with this amount of weight loss includes malignancies, gastrointestinal disorders, endocrine disorders, and infectious diseases. Assuming these disorders are excluded, the most likely diagnosis is avoidant/restrictive food intake disorder (ARFID). Avoidant/restrictive food intake disorder was added to the *Diagnostic and Statistical Manual of Mental Disorders*, Fifth Edition (DSM-5), in 2013. It is characterized by problematic eating habits that place the patient at risk for nutritional deficiencies and weight loss. Avoidant/restrictive food intake disorder is distinct from other eating disorders, such as anorexia nervosa and bulimia nervosa, in that the abnormal eating behaviors in ARFID are not motivated by a disturbance in body image or the desire to be thinner.

EPIDEMIOLOGY

The prevalence of ARFID is estimated to be 3% to 5% among children and adolescents. The population of patients with ARFID is typically younger than the average patient with anorexia nervosa or bulimia nervosa. Avoidant/restrictive food intake disorder is slightly more common in males than in females, which also differs from other eating disorders. Patients with ARFID are more likely to have a comorbid anxiety disorder than a mood disorder.

SIGNS AND SYMPTOMS

According to the DSM-5, ARFID is characterized by heterogeneous and problematic eating habits, which may be related to an intolerance of foods based on texture, taste, or appearance; a fear of potential adverse consequences of eating that are not weight related (e.g., choking or vomiting); and/or an overall lack of interest in food or eating. To meet the diagnostic criteria for ARFID, the patient must demonstrate at least one of the following: (1) significant weight loss (or failure to achieve expected weight gain or faltering growth in children), (2) significant nutritional deficiency, (3) dependence on enteral feeding or oral nutritional supplements, or (4) marked interference with psychosocial functioning.

As in Lucas's case, ARFID may develop after a traumatic food event such as choking or vomiting, such that there is now an aversion to several other foods based on certain shared sensory properties. Lucas first eliminated other meats after choking on a piece of steak, which then progressed to eliminating other solid foods. When due to an adverse incident involving food intake, a change in eating habits is generally acute with a sharp drop in food volume intake.

Signs and symptoms of ARFID may include weight loss, gastrointestinal discomfort, fatigue, dizziness, and syncope, as well as features of more longstanding malnutrition, which include cold intolerance, amenorrhea in females, dry skin, and hair loss. Vital sign abnormalities common in states of malnutrition include orthostatic vital signs, hypotension, hypothermia, and bradycardia in addition to findings of cachexia, scaphoid abdomen, pallor, and lanugo on examination.

ASSESSMENT

A diagnosis of ARFID begins with taking a careful history of eating habits and a medical workup that evaluates for coexisting medical conditions. As mentioned earlier, there is a broad medical differential diagnosis for individuals presenting with these signs and symptoms that includes celiac disease, inflammatory bowel disease, achalasia, hyperthyroidism, Addison's disease, type 1 diabetes, human immunodeficiency virus (HIV), and other eating disorders such as anorexia nervosa and bulimia nervosa.

A thorough psychiatric assessment is critical, as psychiatric comorbidities such as attention-deficit/hyperactivity disorder, generalized anxiety disorder, and OCD may coexist in a patient with ARFID. Formal assessments using the Pica ARFID and Rumination Disorder Interview (PARDI) and the Eating Disorder Examination—ARFID module (EDE-ARFID) may be helpful in establishing a diagnosis of ARFID.

LEVEL OF CARE

The level of care for a patient with ARFID depends on the degree of medical stability, malnutrition, and oral intake. Generally, patients with a current body mass index (BMI) below the 75th percentile of the median BMI for sex and age require an admission to a medical inpatient unit for structured refeeding with close monitoring of electrolyte changes that may indicate refeeding syndrome. Intensive outpatient eating disorder programs or day treatment programs may be considered if the patient has normal vital signs, has normal weight, and is medically stable.

BIOLOGICAL TREATMENT

The primary endpoint of biological treatment is weight gain and weight stabilization, generally through reliance on enteral tube feeding while the patient works closely with a multidisciplinary team including a dietitian, a therapist, and a psychiatrist to achieve greater nutrition via oral intake. Off-label usage of cyproheptadine may be beneficial in a subgroup of patients who present primarily with a lack of interest in food. Cyproheptadine increases appetite and gastric accommodation through antihistaminergic and antiserotonergic mechanisms of action.

At this time, there is no psychopharmacologic treatment approved by the Food and Drug Administration (FDA) for the treatment of ARFID. However, several small studies have investigated the use of olanzapine, mirtazapine, and buspirone, among others, to serve as potential medication treatments of food-related anxiety that may be considered in conjunction with other therapies, which are described next.

PSYCHOSOCIAL TREATMENT

Psychotherapy is a critical part of the treatment of ARFID and must target the underlying reasons for the disorder through the use of desensitization and gradual exposure-based therapy. For these reasons, several studies have incorporated the use of exposure-based cognitive behavioral therapy (CBT) for the treatment of ARFID. The components of CBT for ARFID include psychoeducation, monitoring food intake, implementing regular eating times, adding calories if the child is underweight, gradually increasing food variety, and relapse prevention strategies. When children are trying new foods, they are encouraged to explore a new food slowly, for example, by describing what it looks, feels, smells, and tastes like. Children with ARFID should be encouraged to keep practicing and trying new foods, as it can take 10 or more tries to become comfortable with a new food. Strategies for trying new foods include adding a small portion of a novel food to a preferred food, adding a preferred condiment or spice, trying different presentations of novel foods (e.g., cooked versus raw), and deconstructing a new food into its component parts. Cognitive behavioral therapy for ARFID also teaches children strategies to recognize hunger cues and increase their enjoyment of eating. Relapse prevention strategies include noting how the child's eating has improved, thinking about future triggers for relapse, knowing how to identify signs of a relapse, and deciding which CBT techniques to continue practicing. Overall, approaches involving multidisciplinary teams composed of dietitians, pediatricians, psychiatrists, and psychologists have been shown to be most effective in treating ARFID.

KEY POINTS TO REMEMBER

- Avoidant/restrictive food intake disorder is a relatively new diagnosis introduced in the DSM-5 that is characterized by food avoidance relating to lack of interest, fear, or sensory aversion.
- Compared to other eating disorders, ARFID is more likely to present in younger males with a median age of 11 to 12 years.
- Unlike patients with anorexia nervosa and bulimia nervosa, patients with ARFID are not motivated by a disturbance in body image.
- Successful treatment plans employ a multidisciplinary approach that includes medical and psychotherapeutic interventions.

Further Reading

Bourne L, Bryant-Waugh R, Cook J, et al. Avoidant/restrictive food intake disorder: A systematic scoping review of the current literature. *Psychiatry Res* 2020;288:112961.

Brigham KS, Manzo LD, Eddy KT, et al. Evaluation and treatment of avoidant/restrictive food intake disorder (ARFID) in adolescents. *Curr Pediatr Rep* 2018;6(2):107–113.

Bryant-Waugh R, Micali N, Cooke L, et al. Development of the Pica, ARFID, and Rumination Disorder Interview, a multi-informant, semi-structured interview of feeding disorders across the lifespan: A pilot study for ages 10–22. *Int J Eat Disord* 2019;52(4):378–387.

Keery H, LeMay-Russell S, Barnes TL, et al. Attributes of children and adolescents with avoidant/restrictive food intake disorder. *J Eat Disord* 2019;7:31.

Nicely TA, Lane-Loney S, Masciulli E, et al. Prevalence and characteristics of avoidant/restrictive food intake disorder in a cohort of young patients in day treatment for eating disorders. *J Eat Disord* 2014;2(1):21.

Zickgraf HF, Ellis JM. Initial validation of the nine-item avoidant/restrictive food intake disorder screen (NIAS): A measure of three restrictive eating patterns. *Appetite* 2018;123:32–42.

Zimmerman J, Fisher M. Avoidant/restrictive food intake disorder (ARFID). *Curr Probl Pediatr Adolesc Health Care* 2017;47(4):95–103.

23 A teenage girl with low body mass index due to restricting food intake

Kathryn S. Czepiel

Ellen is a healthy, 19-year-old female and a sophomore at a prestigious college. She presents for a routine physical examination. She has been a patient of yours since she was in elementary school. You notice that her face appears thinner compared to when you last saw her, and her clothes have a baggy fit. Her growth chart confirms this showing a significant drop in weight with an associated drop and body mass index (BMI) from 20 to 16.5 kg/m^2 in the last year.

Ellen is a high-achieving student athlete on the collegiate cross-country ski team with a 4.0 grade point average. Ellen's mom reports that she's been training harder during this season to prepare for competition and manage her stress levels. Ellen has started running daily and has cut out fast-food item and all sweets from her diet. You ask Ellen how she feels about her body. She admits she's lost some weight but denies body image or weight concerns.

What Do You Do Now?

You are concerned that Ellen may have an eating disorder such as anorexia nervosa (AN). It is not atypical for patients with AN to deny weight concerns. Given this degree of unexpected weight loss and deviation in her growth curve, it would be appropriate to consider referring Ellen for a psychiatric evaluation after openly discussing your concerns about her health. It would be helpful to approach this topic using motivational interviewing that is both empathetic and validating. Additionally, it is important to assess for vital sign abnormalities, electrolyte derangements, and suicidality to assess her need for more immediate medical attention.

EPIDEMIOLOGY

Anorexia nervosa has a prevalence of 1% to 2% among females in the United States, with 0.3% to 0.7% of teenage girls affected. The typical age of onset is mid- to late adolescence (14 to 18 years). Prepubertal onset is less common. Younger age of onset is associated with improved prognosis. Ninety-two percent of affected individuals are female, and AN is less common among Hispanic and non-Hispanic Black populations than Caucasians. Suicide risk is elevated in patients with AN with an 18 times higher risk compared to patients without AN. The most common psychiatric comorbidities are major depressive disorder (MDD) (50%), obsessive-compulsive disorder (OCD) (30%), and Cluster C personality disorders. Common personality traits include perfectionism and harm avoidance. Anorexia nervosa carries the highest mortality rate of any psychiatric illness, where 5% to 18% of patients die from the disorder. Fifty percent of deaths are due to suicide, whereas 50% are due to medical complications.

SIGNS AND SYMPTOMS

According to the *Diagnostic and Statistical Manual of Mental Disorders*, Fifth Edition (DSM-5), three criteria are required for a diagnosis of AN: (1) restriction of energy intake relative to requirements leading to a significantly low body weight in the context of age, sex, developmental trajectory, and physical health; (2) an intense fear of gaining weight or becoming fat, or persistent behavior that interferes with weight gain, even though at a significantly low weight; and (3) disturbance in the way in which one's body weight or shape is experienced, undue influence of body weight or shape on self-evaluation, or persistent lack of recognition of the seriousness of the current low body weight.

There are two recognized subtypes of AN: (1) restricting type and (2) binge-eating/purging type. A patient with AN, restricting type experiences weight loss through dieting, fasting, and/or excessive exercise and has not engaged in recurrent episodes of binge eating or purging in the prior three months. In comparison, a patient with AN, binge-eating/purging type has engaged in recurrent episodes of binge-eating or purging behavior within the past three months. Purging behaviors may include self-induced vomiting, as well as diuretic or laxative misuse. The severity of AN is defined by deviation from the normal BMI, ranging from mildly severe low body weight (BMI ≥17) to extremely severe low body weight (BMI <15). Ellen meets criteria for moderately severe low body weight with a BMI of 16.5.

ASSESSMENT

When assessing a patient with suspected AN, it is important to obtain a history from multiple sources, as many patients will attempt to conceal their efforts to lose weight and minimize their symptoms. Parents may also be unaware of many eating disorder–related behaviors. Screening tools such as the "Sick, Control, One, Fat, Food" (SCOFF) questionnaire or the Eating Disorders Diagnostic Scale may be helpful to identify eating disorders in adolescents. The SCOFF questionnaire is a five-item screening measure to assess for the presence of an eating disorder. It is important to determine the onset and course of the eating disorder, highest and lowest weight, and the patient's desired weight. The clinician should inquire about the use of laxatives, diuretics, or diet pills. A detailed interview may reveal a history of progressive weight loss, reduced intake of high-calorie foods, excessive exercise habits, and dissatisfaction with one's body shape that results in low self-esteem and frequent body checking. Amenorrhea is also common among females with AN.

As part of the initial assessment of a patient with AN, it is critical to complete a thorough medical assessment and physical examination that include a review of vital signs with attention to blood pressure, heart rate, and body temperature, all of which can be abnormally low in patients with AN. The physical examination and laboratory studies should seek to exclude medical causes for weight loss (e.g., hyperthyroidism, gastrointestinal illness, malignancy, or chronic infection), malnutrition, and substance use. Findings on physical examination that are common among individuals with AN are cachexia, dry skin, hair loss, and lanugo. Features predominant in AN, binge-eating/purging subtype include erosion of tooth enamel and hypertrophied salivary glands. The medical assessment should also assess for common medical complications of AN including arrhythmia, hypotension, bradycardia, amenorrhea, osteoporosis, dehydration, constipation, and impaired fertility. Recurrent vomiting can also result in gastritis, pancreatitis, and esophagitis. The mental status examination of a patient with suspected AN should include a brief cognitive exam. Common findings include impaired set-shifting ability and perceptual abilities.

Laboratory studies may reveal decreased sodium, potassium, chloride, calcium, magnesium, and phosphorus levels, with rises in bicarbonate, cholesterol, liver enzymes, and amylase. Decreases in all blood cell types (leukopenia, anemia, thrombocytopenia) and low serum albumin may also be present. In severe forms of malnutrition, an electrocardiogram (EKG) may reveal bradycardia with prolongation of the QTc interval.

LEVEL OF CARE

International clinical guidelines agree that outpatient therapy is consistently recommended as the first-line treatment for patients with AN. Immediate medical hospitalization is warranted in patients with a BMI <15, unstable vital signs, growth arrest or pubertal delay, evidence of dehydration, life-threatening electrolyte derangements, acute refusal to eat, suicidality, or prior failure of outpatient care. The inpatient medical admission is focused on safe refeeding and weight gain aimed at 0.5 to 1.5 kilograms per week under close medical supervision. Tube feeding should be considered only in cases of medical instability. A transfer from inpatient to residential or day treatment programs is appropriate once the patient has been medically stabilized. Regardless of the level of care, a multidisciplinary approach to treatment involving a pediatric dietician, pediatrician, psychologist, psychiatrist, and family therapist is essential.

BIOLOGICAL TREATMENT

Pharmacotherapy, including antidepressant and antipsychotic medications, should not be used as the primary treatment for patients with AN. While no medications have consistently demonstrated efficacy for weight gain in AN, atypical antipsychotics, such as olanzapine, have shown the most promise. If antipsychotics are used in this population, the potential for side effects, particularly cardiac side effects and prolongation of the QTc interval, must be monitored closely. It is important to note that the symptoms of comorbid MDD and OCD may resolve with weight gain alone.

It is generally recommended that patients receive adequate calcium intake, as well as vitamin D supplementation. Recommendations for the treatment of osteoporosis and bone loss in patients with AN are still evolving. There is emerging evidence that transdermal estrogen, as opposed to oral contraceptives that suppress insulin-like growth factor 1, may be effective in improving bone mass.

PSYCHOSOCIAL TREATMENT

Patients with AN are generally ambivalent about change and therefore benefit from psychotherapy during both the acute and maintenance phases of treatment. Family-based treatment (Maudsley family therapy) is the first-line treatment for AN in adolescents. Five randomized controlled trials have been completed showing the efficacy of this treatment. Family-based treatment programs are designed with three distinct treatment phases spread over a six- to 12-month period. Phase one of family-based treatment is the weight restoration phase and typically lasts for at least three months. In this phase of treatment, the focus is helping the patient to achieve weight gain. A major theme of this phase is helping the parents and adolescent to "externalize" the disorder and accept that the adolescent's eating disorder behaviors are beyond their control. Parents are coached to set the clear expectation that the adolescent gain weight. In this phase of treatment, the patient and parents eat all meals together as a family. Parents are responsible for preparing the adolescent's meals and the patient is not permitted to choose the amount or type of food they eat. Phase two of treatment begins once the adolescent is eating with the family on a regular basis and with minimal resistance. During this phase of treatment, the adolescent gradually begins to eat meals away from their parents with developmentally appropriate eating being the target. In phase three, the goal is return to normal development. This phase is initiated when the adolescent is maintaining weight above 95% of their ideal body weight. The patient eats most meals on their own and selects foods independently. Parents remain vigilant for signs of relapse, while allowing the patient to establish a healthy adolescent identity.

While no specific individual psychotherapies for AN have demonstrated superiority over supportive psychotherapy, individual psychotherapy may play an important adjunctive role in treatment, particularly once weight restoration has been achieved. Cognitive behavioral therapy (CBT) for AN has demonstrated inconsistent results in the treatment of AN in adolescents and is mostly beneficial for treating the body shape perceptions that maintain the disorder. Psychodynamic psychotherapy for AN focuses on improving self-efficacy, self-esteem, and insight to maintain recovery.

The American Academy of Child and Adolescent Psychiatry (AACAP) has published a Facts for Families article on eating disorders, which contains helpful information for parents and caregivers (https://www.aacap.org/AACAP/Families_and_Youth/Facts_for_Families/FFF-Guide/Teenagers-With-Eating-Disorders-2.aspx).

KEY POINTS TO REMEMBER

- Anorexia nervosa is an eating disorder defined by two subtypes, restricting and binge eating/purging, that presents with low body weight, fear of weight gain, and disturbed body image.
- Be mindful of electrolyte derangements that include decreased sodium, potassium, chloride, calcium, magnesium, and phosphorus levels, some of which can worsen significantly with refeeding.
- Pharmacotherapy should not be the primary treatment for AN.
- Psychotherapy with family-based therapy is the gold standard treatment option for children and adolescents with the disorder.

Further Reading

Hilbert A, Hoek HW, Schmidt R. Evidence-based clinical guidelines for eating disorders: International comparison. *Curr Opin Psychiatry* 2017;30(6):423–437.

Lock J, La Via MC, American Academy of Child and Adolescent Psychiatry Committee on Quality Improvement. Practice parameter for the assessment and treatment of children and adolescents with eating disorders. *J Am Acad Child Adolesc Psychiatry* 2015;54(5):412–425.

Mitchell JE, Peterson CB. Anorexia nervosa. *N Engl J Med* 2020;382(14):1343–1351.

National Institute for Health and Care Excellence. *Eating Disorders: Recognition and Treatment. Clinical Guidelines*. London: National Institute for Health and Care Excellence, 2017.

Resmark G, Herpertz S, Herpertz-Dahlmann B, et al. Treatment of anorexia nervosa: New evidence-based guidelines. *J Clin Med* 2019;8(2):153.

24 Recurrent episodes of binging and purging

Christina L. Macenski

A 16-year-old girl presents to the pediatrician with her father for an annual wellness visit. She reports school is going well and her father proudly shares that she is a straight A student who was recently elected class president. She enjoys playing softball and has a group of close friends whom she spends time with on weekends. When asked about her diet, her father voices frustration that she refuses to eat dinner with the family and often brings large quantities of food to her room to eat alone. He has tried several times to persuade her to eat with the family without success and attributes this behavior to "teenage angst." The patient avoids eye contact during this discussion. When interviewed alone, she becomes tearful and states, "I don't want to eat dinner with my family because I lose control and eat too much, even though I am already overweight." She admits to vomiting after dinner if she overeats to keep her weight down. Physical examination is notable for a body mass index (BMI) of 22 and scarring on the dorsum of her knuckles (Russell's sign). She denies any symptoms of depression, suicidal ideation, or self-harm behaviors.

What Do You Do Now?

The patient is suffering from bulimia nervosa (BN), an eating disorder characterized by episodes of binge eating followed by excessive compensatory behaviors to prevent weight gain. Bulimia nervosa can follow an acute, episodic, or chronic course and has high rates of relapse (~50% at five years). While data regarding the effects of early diagnosis and intervention are lacking in both children and adults, there is evidence that the duration of untreated illness is inversely related to rate of recovery.

EPIDEMIOLOGY

The lifetime prevalence of BN among adolescents has been estimated to range from 0.8% to 1.7%. It should be noted that this estimate does not include individuals with subthreshold or atypical eating disorders, which may share similarities with BN. Eating disorders, as a whole, are 10 times more common in girls than in boys. Bulimia nervosa typically presents in late adolescence or young adulthood, which may account for the higher lifetime prevalence of BN in adults, which is estimated at 0.9% to 3%. Risk factors for the development of BN include genetics (heritability 28% to 83%), parental factors such as mental illness or rigid views on weight gain, and patient variables such as low self-esteem, depression, social anxiety, or history of childhood trauma. Patients with a premorbid history of obesity may also be at increased risk for developing BN. The severity of comorbid psychiatric disease predicts worse long-term outcomes.

SIGNS AND SYMPTOMS

According to the *Diagnostic and Statistical Manual of Mental Disorders*, Fifth Edition (DSM-5), BN is characterized by recurrent episodes of binge eating along with recurrent inappropriate compensatory behaviors to prevent weight gain (e.g., self-induced vomiting, fasting, excessive exercise, laxative or diuretic misuse) at least once per week for three months. Binge eating is defined as (1) eating an amount of food that is definitely larger than what most individuals would eat under similar circumstances in a discrete time period and (2) a sense of lack of control over eating during the episode. In addition, a patient's self-evaluation must be unduly affected by weight and body shape concerns. Meeting full criteria for anorexia nervosa is an exclusionary criterion. Specifiers include remission status (partial vs. full) and severity based on number of episodes of inappropriate compensatory behaviors per week, ranging from mild (one to three episodes) to extreme (14 or more). Bulimia nervosa is often clinically divided into purging versus restrictive subtypes, although the DSM-5 makes no such distinction. Patients are typically of normal weight or are overweight; in children and adolescents this is calculated using BMI-for-age rather than standard adult BMI calculations. BMI-for-age greater than the fifth percentile is considered normal as long as children maintain a normal growth trajectory.

Since BN most commonly presents in adolescence and young adulthood, clinical features of adolescent BN are quite similar to adult presentations. However, features of BN that are more common in adolescents include a purging subtype and secretiveness. The use of laxatives, diuretics, and diet pills is less common in the pediatric population. Dieting is a common precursor to BN. Common binge-eating triggers include negative emotions, increased interpersonal stress, dietary restriction, boredom, and negative thoughts related to body image. Binge eating usually provides temporary relief of negative emotions but is followed by self-critical thoughts.

ASSESSMENT

Bulimia nervosa is a clinical diagnosis. While laboratory tests can provide supportive evidence in some cases, they are not required for the diagnosis and are often normal. A thorough history from both the patient and the caregiver is the crux of an effective evaluation and should include eating behavior symptoms, detailed eating patterns with relation to compensatory behaviors, common triggers, comorbid psychiatric disorders, psychosocial stressors, family stressors and supports, and an exploration of the patient's understanding or insight into their illness. It is important to establish a strong therapeutic alliance to accurately monitor eating disorder symptoms and behaviors over time.

On mental status examination, patients with BN are often meticulously dressed and cooperative and exhibit decreased eye contact, depressed affect with or without suicidal ideation, anxious mood/affect, linear thought process, thought content fixated on food or body image, poor judgment (as evidenced by compensatory behaviors), and little insight into their distorted body image. Features of cognition such as attention, concentration, memory, and intellect are typically normal. Several assessment tools have been created to aid in assessing patients with eating disorders, the gold standard being the Eating Disorders Examination (EDE). The EDE evaluates eating disorder symptoms within the last 28 days and is validated for children nine to 18 years old. There is also a younger children's version validated in children seven years and older. Assessment tools should not replace the clinical interview but rather supplement it.

All patients with suspected BN should undergo a complete physical examination with a basic laboratory workup that includes serum electrolytes, blood urea nitrogen, creatinine, thyroid studies, complete blood count, inflammatory markers, liver enzymes, and urinalysis. Additional workup can be considered based on the clinical presentation. While uncommon in BN, those with evidence of severe malnourishment should have special attention paid to serum calcium, magnesium, phosphorus, and ferritin with additional workup including an electrocardiogram. Females with amenorrhea for greater than six months should also undergo dual-energy x-ray absorptiometry for bone density measurements and serum estradiol, luteinizing hormone, and follicle-stimulating hormone to evaluate functioning of the hypothalamic-pituitary-adrenal axis. A toxicology screen can be considered for patients in whom comorbid substance use is suspected. Serum amylase and stool/urine studies (e.g., bisacodyl, emodin, aloe-emodin) can be useful in patients to detect surreptitious vomiting or suspected laxative abuse, respectively.

The differential diagnosis for BN is broad and includes medical causes for binge eating (e.g., Prader-Willi syndrome), other eating disorders, major depressive disorder, and obsessive-compulsive disorder. Mood and anxiety disorders are highly comorbid with BN and all patients should be screened with appropriate measures and clinical interview.

LEVEL OF CARE

Most patients diagnosed with BN are managed in the outpatient setting. However, there are higher levels of care available such as intensive outpatient treatment, partial hospitalization, residential treatment, and inpatient hospitalization. Generally, medical inpatient hospitalization for any eating disorder is reserved for children and adolescents with medical instability. Patients with BN are unlikely to meet criteria for medical instability, as they are typically of normal weight and less malnourished. Level-of-care determinations should also take into account motivation to recover, fixation on maladaptive thoughts, cooperation with treatment, needed structure or supervision to ensure recovery, comorbid psychiatric disorders, suicidality, substance use, psychosocial stressors, social supports, and prior responses to treatment.

BIOLOGICAL TREATMENT

Fluoxetine, a selective serotonin reuptake inhibitor (SSRI), is the only Food and Drug Administration (FDA)-approved medication for the treatment of BN in adults. It should be noted that there are no FDA-approved medications for BN in children; however, fluoxetine and other antidepressants are commonly used in clinical practice to treat patients under 18 years of age. Antidepressants have been shown to reduce the core symptoms of binge eating and compensatory vomiting while also improving the anxiety associated with the disorder. Patients with comorbid depression or anxiety who meet full criteria for the DSM-5 disorder may especially benefit from treatment with an antidepressant. Selective serotonin reuptake inhibitors are preferred over other antidepressants such as tricyclic antidepressants or monoamine oxidase inhibitors due to a more favorable side effect and toxicity profile. Bupropion, a norepinephrine and dopamine reuptake inhibitor, is contraindicated due to increased risk of seizures in patients with eating disorders. Selective serotonin reuptake inhibitors are typically prescribed at higher doses for BN (the FDA-approved dose for adults is 60 mg per day), which may cause increased side effects such as constipation, nausea, insomnia, and sexual dysfunction, which is particularly problematic in adolescents, who are at high risk for nonadherence. In children and adolescents, it is also important to educate patients and families about the FDA black-box warning concerning increased suicidality associated with SSRIs.

Other medications such as topiramate, ondansetron, and mood stabilizers have been used to treat adult patients with BN. Topiramate has been shown to reduce binge/purge days but is limited by side effects including weight loss and cognitive disturbances. Ondansetron has been shown to reduce binge/purge frequency in several small studies. Patients with comorbid bipolar disorder may benefit from a mood stabilizer, although lithium and valproic can both lead to weight gain, which is problematic for adherence. Additionally, maintaining stable lithium levels is challenging in patients with disordered eating. The use of antipsychotics is similarly limited due to their side effect of weight gain. The decision to trial these medications in children is typically made on a case-by-case basis.

Finally, lisdexamfetamine, a stimulant medication, has been FDA approved for the treatment of binge-eating disorder in adults. Given the similarities between binge-eating disorder and BN, clinical trials of lisdexamfetamine for the treatment of BN are currently underway.

PSYCHOSOCIAL TREATMENT

The goals of treatment for BN are to eliminate the binge-purge cycle, establish healthy eating habits, maintain a healthy body weight, and minimize restrictive eating patterns. Treatment begins with psychoeducation about the signs and symptoms of the illness and treatment options. The American Academy of Child and Adolescent Psychiatry (AACAP) has published a Facts for Families article, which can be distributed to parents and caregivers (https://www.aacap.org/AACAP/Families_and_Youth/Facts_for_Families/ FFF-Guide/Teenagers-With-Eating-Disorders-2.aspx). A nutritional consultation is an essential early component of treatment and should focus on initiating regular eating behavior patterns without binging, ceasing excessive compensatory behaviors, correcting nutritional deficits, and encouraging healthy exercise. Maintaining optimal weight is important, as deviance from this may contribute to disordered eating behaviors. The treatment of BN requires a multidisciplinary approach with a team consisting of psychiatrists, dentists, pediatricians, psychologists, family therapists, dieticians, school staff, and social workers to provide comprehensive support.

Psychotherapy has been shown to be effective in patients with BN, specifically cognitive behavioral therapy (CBT) and family therapy. Cognitive behavioral therapy is most effective when focused on eating disorder symptoms and maladaptive thoughts. It can be used to help the patient learn non-food-related, more adaptive coping skills to manage distress and solve problems. Family therapy is particularly helpful for children and adolescents, as home dynamics can be a significant source of stress. Supportive, interpersonal, psychodynamic, and group psychotherapy can also be considered, although evidence of their effectiveness in BN is not as robust.

KEY POINTS TO REMEMBER

- Bulimia nervosa is an eating disorder characterized by episodes of binging with associated compensatory behaviors that can include vomiting, fasting, excessive exercise, and laxative or diuretic abuse.
- Bulimia nervosa is a clinical diagnosis and physical examination/laboratory findings are typically normal.
- Pediatric patients with BN are of normal or increased weight, which can be determined by calculating a BMI-for-age greater than the fifth percentile.
- The mainstay for treatment of pediatric BN includes SSRIs and psychotherapy (CBT and/or family therapy).
- A multidisciplinary approach to the treatment of BN is associated with better outcomes and should include psychiatrists, dentists, pediatricians, psychologists, family therapists, dieticians, school staff, and social workers.

Further Reading

American Psychiatric Association. *Treating Eating Disorders: A Quick Reference Guide. American Psychiatric Association Practice Guidelines for the Treatment of Psychiatric Disorders: Compendium 2006.* Washington, DC: American Psychiatric Association, 2006:224–252.

Couturier J, Lock J. A review of medication use for children and adolescents with eating disorders. *J Can Acad Child Adolesc Psychiatry* 2007;16(4):173.

Le Grange D, Crosby RD, Rathouz PJ, et al. A randomized controlled comparison of family-based treatment and supportive psychotherapy for adolescent bulimia nervosa. *Arch Gen Psychiatry* 2007;64(9):1049–1056.

Le Grange D, Lock J, Agras WS, et al. Randomized clinical trial of family-based treatment and cognitive-behavioral therapy for adolescent bulimia nervosa. *J Am Acad Child Adolesc Psychiatry* 2015;54(11):886–894.

Mairs R, Nicholls D. Assessment and treatment of eating disorders in children and adolescents. *Arch Dis Child* 2016;101(12):1168–1175.

Schmidt U, Brown A, McClelland J, et al. Will a comprehensive, person-centered, team-based early intervention approach to first episode illness improve outcomes in eating disorders? *Int J Eat Disord* 2016;49(4):374–377.

Smink FR, van Hoeken D, Oldehinkel AJ, et al. Prevalence and severity of DSM-5 eating disorders in a community cohort of adolescents. *Int J Eat Disord* 2014;47(6):610–619.

25 A young boy with stool soiling

Kathryn S. Czepiel

Charlie is a six-year-old boy who presents for his annual physical. His mother reports he has been stooling himself a few times per week. She describes finding watery, loose stools in his underwear. She is worried that Charlie ignores the stools and denies having stooled himself. She explains that this started when he began kindergarten a few weeks ago. Last week, Charlie was playing with his cousins when he had an accident. His teacher reports this is also happening at school. His classmates tease Charlie about how he smells. Charlie did not have problems with potty training and seems to stool regularly at home. His stools are occasionally so large that they clog the toilet.

Charlie's physical examination reveals palpable masses in the left lower quadrant of his abdomen. His abdomen is otherwise soft and nontender. There are no visible rashes. When asked about using the toilet, Charlie explains that he is scared of using the toilets at school.

What Do You Do Now?

Charlie is suffering from functional encopresis, an elimination disorder in which an individual has repeated passage of feces into inappropriate places (e.g., clothing, floor) that is not due to an organic illness. The most common reason for functional encopresis is constipation with overflow incontinence.

EPIDEMIOLOGY

Functional encopresis is most common in children between five and 10 years of age, with prevalence rates ranging between 1.5% and 7.5% among children. The prevalence of encopresis decreases with age and rarely affects adolescents. Boys are three to six times more likely to be affected by encopresis than girls. Encopresis makes up about a quarter of pediatric gastroenterology visits and 3% to 6% of pediatric psychiatry referrals. About one-quarter of children with functional encopresis also have functional enuresis.

The constipation underlying encopresis often begins with episodes of stool withholding. Stool withholding involves voluntary contraction of the external anal sphincter that delays passage of feces beyond the rectosigmoid colon. Stools usually contain about 75% water; however, the longer the stool is retained, the more water is absorbed, making the stools harder and more painful to pass. Chronic stool withholding can stretch colonic walls and interfere with neuronal activity, such that children no longer respond to normal sensations prompting defecation. This results in larger stools with impacted fecal matter that may leak out as liquid stools, causing fecal soiling. Unfortunately, this creates a vicious cycle of further stool withholding to avoid passing large, painful stools.

SIGNS AND SYMPTOMS

According to the *Diagnostic and Statistical Manual of Mental Disorders*, Fifth Edition (DSM-5), encopresis is characterized by repeated passage of feces into inappropriate places that is either intentional or involuntary, occurring at least once monthly for at least three months. The behavior is not attributable to the physiological effects of a substance such as laxatives or another medical condition other than constipation. The individual must be at least four years of age (or equivalent developmental level). Signs and symptoms of encopresis can include occasional passage of very large stools, secretive behavior associated with bowel movements, fecal incontinence, and passage of very hard stools.

ASSESSMENT

The majority of encopresis is functional, where only 5% to 10% of chronic encopresis cases are related to organic fecal incontinence. In making the diagnosis of encopresis, it is essential to characterize whether there is evidence of underlying constipation and overflow incontinence. Psychosocial effects of functional encopresis among school-aged children include teasing and bullying by peers related to fecal soiling. In a child such as Charlie with repeated soiling episodes, it is not uncommon for children to develop olfactory adaptation, such that they are no longer sensitive to the odor of feces, making them less likely to detect accidents.

A detailed medical history and physical examination are essential to differentiate between functional encopresis and organic encopresis. It is best to organize the medical history based on the perinatal and developmental history, current stooling patterns, and preceding contextual history. The perinatal and developmental history should include questions about the neonatal passage of meconium and potty-training history with attention to the age of fecal continence. The patient's current stooling patterns including frequency of stools, timing and location of stools, size of stools, and volume of accidentally passed stools should be determined. Finally, contextual history questions should inquire about triggering events including transitions (e.g., starting a new school, change in caregivers) and the possibility of trauma or abuse.

These questions help to narrow the differential diagnosis between functional and organic causes for encopresis. The differential diagnosis for organic causes of encopresis includes anatomic (e.g., imperforate anus, ectopic anus, anal stenosis, or history of bowel resection), neurologic (e.g., Hirschsprung disease, neuronal intestinal dysplasia, Chagas disease, or spinal cord injury), metabolic (e.g., hypothyroidism, hypoparathyroidism, chronic diabetes leading to intestinal pseudo-obstruction, pheochromocytoma causing nonretentive encopresis, celiac disease), and iatrogenic (e.g., laxative or diuretic overuse, tricyclic antidepressants or iron causing constipation).

The psychiatric assessment of a child with encopresis should assess for associated psychiatric disorders that may contribute to fecal soiling. For example, children with anxiety disorders may avoid using the toilet, while children with attention-deficit/hyperactivity disorder (ADHD) may be too distractible to use the toilet or may be prone to constipation because of insufficient time spent on the toilet. Finally, children with oppositional defiant disorder (ODD), with conduct disorder, or experiencing abuse may soil themselves willfully.

PREVENTION

Prevention of functional encopresis is focused on preventing constipation. Children should be encouraged to have regular physical activity and frequent toilet time, especially during times of childhood transition when they may be at the highest risk of toilet avoidance. High fiber and high fluid intake are additional components of maintaining regular bowel movements.

BIOLOGICAL TREATMENT

If left untreated, encopresis can progress to enuresis, frequent urinary tract infections, rectal prolapse, and pelvic dyssynergia (lack of coordination of pelvic floor muscles). Organic encopresis generally resolves with treatment of the underlying etiology. Functional encopresis is so often a result of stool withholding secondary to constipation that it is essential to first treat the underlying constipation. This is generally initiated by the child's pediatrician. Helping the child to pass soft fecal matter without associated pain will help break the cycle of withholding. A referral to a pediatric gastroenterologist is recommended when efforts toward treating constipation have been unsuccessful for greater than six months. Laxatives including a variety of osmotic agents, stimulants, and lubricating agents may be used. Dietary modifications including increased fluid and fiber intake are of unclear effectiveness in treating children with known constipation, though these should be emphasized as part of maintenance therapy once a patient is having one to two soft stools daily.

PSYCHOSOCIAL TREATMENT

Functional encopresis with constipation and fecal overflow, as in Charlie's case, is best treated with a multidisciplinary approach. The psychosocial approach to treating this disorder relies on behavioral modification that includes operant conditioning. While positive reinforcement systems should focus on improving the patient's cooperation and not solely on proper elimination, specific behavioral targets may vary based on the child's age and interests. Caregivers play an important role in treatment, and psychoeducation about the disorder is an important component of treatment. The American Academy of Child and Adolescent Psychiatry (AACAP) has published a Facts for Families article, which contains helpful information (https://www.aacap.org/AACAP/Families_and_Youth/Facts_for_Families/FFF-Guide/Problems-With-Soiling-and-Bowel-Control-048.aspx). Caregivers may play a part in toilet desensitization with gradually progressive toilet exposures, both in private and public restrooms, through gradually increasing time spent sitting on the toilet. Children frequently respond well to toilet time if it is associated with special toys such as books or hand-held electronics that are otherwise not available to them.

> **KEY POINTS TO REMEMBER**
>
> · Over 90% of cases of pediatric encopresis are due to functional stool withholding. The most common cause of functional encopresis is constipation.
> · Psychiatric disorders that can contribute to functional encopresis include anxiety disorders, ADHD, posttraumatic stress disorder, ODD, and conduct disorder.
> · Functional encopresis is most common in children between five and 10 years of age at points of transition (e.g., breast milk to solid food, school enrollment).
> · Hallmarks of encopresis include repeated passage of feces in inappropriate locations in an individual older than four years of age.
> · Treatment of the underlying etiology, whether constipation or another organic cause, and behavioral modification make up the cornerstones of management.

Further Reading

Call NA, Mevers JL, McElhanon BO, et al. A multidisciplinary treatment for encopresis in children with developmental disabilities. *J Appl Behav Anal* 2017;50(2):332–344.

Colombo JM, Wassom MC, Rosen JM. Constipation and encopresis in childhood. *Pediatr Rev* 2015;36(9):392–401; quiz 2.

Har AF, Croffie JM. Encopresis. *Pediatr Rev* 2010;31(9):368–374; quiz 74.

McGrath ML, Mellon MW, Murphy L. Empirically supported treatments in pediatric psychology: Constipation and encopresis. *J Pediatr Psychol* 2000;25(4):225–254; discussion 55–56.

Shepard JA, Poler JE Jr, Grabman JH. Evidence-based psychosocial treatments for pediatric elimination disorders. *J Clin Child Adolesc Psychol* 2017;46(6):767–797.

26 An adolescent requesting to pause puberty

Cordelia Y. Ross and
Alex S. Keuroghlian

A 12-year-old child is referred for psychiatric evaluation of depressed mood. The child was assigned female sex at birth yet from an early age insisted on being called by a gender nonbinary name and behaved in a gender-expansive manner, such as expressing interest in traditionally masculine toys and clothing. The parents inform you that their child recently experienced menarche and has requested to talk to an expert about "gender stuff."

On assessment, the patient goes by "Alex" and has "they/them/theirs" (gender nonbinary) pronouns. Alex shares they've been a boy for as long as they can remember and disclosed this to their parents one year ago. Despite being supported in their social gender affirmation (e.g., cutting their hair short, wearing traditional boys' clothing), they have experienced increased disgust about their body and appearance with the onset of puberty. They have learned that there are medications that can pause puberty and they ask if you could prescribe these.

What Do You Do Now?

The patient's presentation is consistent with gender dysphoria, distress associated with incongruence between a person's experienced gender and the gender traditionally associated with their sex assigned at birth. The diagnosis replaces the outdated and nonaffirming term "gender identity disorder" used in the *Diagnostic and Statistical Manual of Mental Disorders*, Fourth Edition (DSM-IV). Gender dysphoria can be associated with challenges in functioning, particularly in social environments, if a person experiences others' perceptions of and behaviors toward them as nonaffirming. As such, among prepubertal children, increasing age is associated with more behavioral and emotional problems, as gender-expansive self-expression may be less commonly accepted by others and met with ostracism or bullying by peers. This distress can be mitigated, and functioning improved, through supportive, gender-affirming communities and environments, as well as specific social, psychological, legal, medical, and surgical approaches to reduce distress, and treatment of any active psychiatric disorders.

EPIDEMIOLOGY

Epidemiologic data regarding gender diversity and gender dysphoria are difficult to obtain. The prevalence of gender dysphoria is thought to range from 0.005% to 0.014% among adults assigned male sex at birth, and 0.002% to 0.003% among adults assigned female sex at birth, though these are likely underestimates since not all of these people present to specialty clinical practices where data is collected. Recent studies suggest that the prevalence of self-reported transgender and gender-diverse identities among children, adolescents, and adults ranges from 0.5% to 1.3%, with an estimated one million adults identifying as transgender in the United States. Based on existing studies utilizing parent report on the Child Behavior Checklist (CBCL), children assigned male sex at birth have been more frequently referred to specialized gender identity clinics until recently. With decreasing societal stigma, greater acceptance of gender diversity, and increased public awareness about gender affirmation options for children, gender specialty clinics in recent years have seen a steady increase in youth referrals.

Psychiatric problems that may be present among children with gender dysphoria include emotional and behavioral difficulties (e.g., anxiety disorders; disruptive, impulse control, and conduct disorders; and major depressive disorder [MDD]). Adolescents and adults with gender dysphoria may suffer from anxiety disorders and MDD. Some reporting has suggested that autism spectrum disorder (ASD) may be more prevalent among clinically referred adolescents with gender dysphoria. While ASD and gender dysphoria may co-occur, social impairments among some adolescents have been considered secondary to other psychiatric disorders and gender minority stress, representing reversible etiologies rather than true ASD. Gender diversity is associated with high levels of discrimination and victimization, leading to poor self-esteem, increased incidence of psychiatric disorders (particularly MDD and anxiety disorders), suicide attempts, school discontinuation, unemployment, and homelessness.

SIGNS AND SYMPTOMS

The *Diagnostic and Statistical Manual of Mental Disorders*, Fifth Edition (DSM-5), distinguishes gender dysphoria in children from that in adolescents and adults. For both groups, diagnostic criteria include symptoms that last for at least six months. Among adults, gender dysphoria involves an incongruence between one's experienced/expressed gender and assigned gender, along with significant distress and problems functioning. The DSM-5 also requires at least two of the following diagnostic criteria: a marked incongruence between one's experienced/expressed gender and primary and/or secondary sex characteristics, a strong desire to be rid of one's primary and/or secondary sex characteristics, a strong desire for primary and/or secondary sex characteristics not traditionally associated with the sex assigned at birth, a strong desire to be of a gender not traditionally associated with the sex assigned birth, a strong desire to be treated as a gender not traditionally associated with the sex assigned at birth, and a strong conviction that one has the typical feelings and reactions of a gender not traditionally associated with the sex assigned at birth.

In children, at least six of the following must be present: a strong desire to be or insistence that one is of a gender not traditionally associated with the sex assigned at birth; a strong preference for wearing clothes typical of a gender not traditionally associated with the sex assigned at birth; a strong preference for gender-expansive roles in play; a strong preference for toys, games, or activities not stereotypically associated with the sex assigned at birth; a strong preference for playmates of a gender not traditionally associated with the patient's sex assigned at birth; a strong rejection of toys, games, or activities traditionally associated with the sex assigned at birth; a strong dislike of one's sexual anatomy; and a strong desire for physical sex characteristics matching one's experienced gender.

Importantly, the very existence of a gender dysphoria diagnosis in the DSM-5 is highly controversial. Many transgender and gender-diverse community advocates have called for removal of this diagnosis, with a shift for billing purposes toward nondiagnosis codes that refer to "factors influencing health status" and billing for services without attaching a diagnosis (e.g., "gender-affirming counseling in childhood" or "psychiatric evaluation preceding gender-affirming surgical intervention"). These proposed diagnostic changes would avoid assuming pathology or distress related to gender diversity and further stigmatizing transgender and gender-diverse people.

Children may demonstrate gender-expansive behaviors as young as ages two to four years, coinciding with when children typically express gendered behaviors and interests. Gender-expansive behavior is common in childhood and may not necessarily warrant clinical intervention. Gender-expansive behavior that is more persistent, insistent, and consistent, and associated with distress, may indicate a need for proactive gender-affirming care.

DEFINITIONS

Gender identity is a person's identification as a girl/woman, boy/man, something else, or having no gender; it refers to one's deeply held core sense of gender, which may not always correspond based on societal expectations to the sex assigned at birth. *Transgender* refers to individuals who identify as a gender not traditionally associated with their sex assigned at birth, while *cisgender* refers to people for whom gender identity corresponds in a traditional way with their sex assigned at birth. *Gender expression* refers to the outward communication of gender; it may include mannerisms, voice, and clothing, and it often does not correspond with or predict gender identity based on societal gender-related notions. *Gender affirmation* is the process by which a person receives care, support, and treatment that validate their gender identity. Gender identity is not the same as *sexual orientation*, which refers to physical, emotional, and romantic attachments to other people. *Gender minority* is an umbrella term that encompasses persons for whom gender identity does not correspond in a traditional way with their sex assigned at birth.

ASSESSMENT

There are no broadly accepted rating scales or tests for gender dysphoria. Clinicians cannot determine through observation of gender expression if a child is or is not transgender or gender diverse, as gender identity is only self-determined and self-declared by patients themselves. Rather, clinicians ought to focus on reducing the child's internal distress related to familial, community, and societal stigma; supporting the child throughout their gender affirmation process; and helping families adopt an accepting and nurturing response to their child's gender-diverse identity. Obtaining detailed and relevant information from the child, and, when the child consents, from the child's parent(s)/caregiver(s), about the child's developmental history of gender-expansive identification and expression will help inform thoughtful clinical formulation and responsive care. Psychiatrists can also help with the assessment and management of any psychiatric disorders and with facilitating referral to pediatric specialists who can assess the need for potential pubertal suppression or gender-affirming hormone therapy, which include pediatric endocrinologists and, increasingly, primary care pediatricians. Clinicians should never presume an individual's gender identity and should work to develop an inclusive understanding of gender identity beyond the traditional binary gender paradigm of girls/women or boys/men.

BIOLOGICAL TREATMENT

The foundational principle in caring for transgender and gender-diverse children and adolescents is affirmation of their gender identity. Gender affirmation processes can include psychological, social, legal, and biological interventions. Biological interventions include pubertal suppression, gender-affirming hormone therapy, and gender-affirming surgery. During

Tanner Stage II, which typically occurs between nine and 11 years of age, a transgender or gender-diverse adolescent may have the option to access pubertal suppression, in which a gonadotropin-releasing hormone (GnRH) analog prevents further development of secondary sex characteristics. Use of GnRH analogs to suppress puberty may avert negative social and emotional consequences of gender dysphoria. Compared to psychosocial support alone, pubertal suppression has been associated with improved internalizing psychopathology and greater improvement in general functioning, as measured by the Children's Global Assessment Scale. Furthermore, those who accessed pubertal suppression versus those who desired it but did not access it had a lower likelihood of suicidal ideation. It is important to highlight that allowing endogenous puberty to occur in a transgender or gender-diverse patient is not a neutral act and may cause serious harm. Withholding gender-affirming medical care may lead to worsening distress, stigmatization, and abuse. Pubertal suppression can also be helpful in extending the exploratory phase for young people who are trying to understand their gender identity.

As early as age 14 years, people may consider the use of gender-affirming hormone therapy (e.g., estradiol or testosterone) to assist with the development of secondary sex characteristics that align with their gender identity. Gender-affirming hormone therapy is associated with improved internalizing psychopathology and general well-being, as well as decreased suicidality.

The earliest age at which transgender and gender-diverse youth may undergo gender-affirming surgeries in the United States is currently evolving, with some procedures now accessible for minors younger than 18 years old. Surgery includes but is not limited to procedures referred to as "top surgery" (e.g., masculine chest construction or breast augmentation) and "bottom surgery" (e.g., phalloplasty or vaginoplasty), as well as chondrolaryngoplasty or "tracheal shave." In some contexts, referral letters from mental health clinicians are currently required to proceed with gender-affirming surgical procedures.

Discontinued Gender Affirmation Experiences

The cessation or reversal of gender affirmation experiences, sometimes referred to as "de-transition," or the possibility of this occurring, may concern the parent(s)/caregiver(s) of transgender and gender-diverse children and adolescents. Data from the United States Transgender Survey (USTS) indicate that 13.1% of transgender and gender-diverse people have experienced past discontinuation of gender affirmation experiences, the great majority of whom cite external factors as the reason for discontinuation (e.g., pressure from a parent, spouse, or employer, or discrimination and harassment from others). Studies suggest that regret after gender affirmation among adolescents who have undergone gender-affirming hormone therapy is virtually zero; regret reported after gonadectomy is 0.3% among adult transgender women and 0.6% among adult transgender men. Approximately 1.9% of adolescents who initiate pubertal suppression discontinue treatment.

PSYCHOSOCIAL TREATMENT

Psychotherapeutic support may be helpful prior to and throughout the gender affirmation process. The goal of therapy is ultimately to help a person explore, discover, and affirm their gender identity, in order to live more comfortably within their gender and body, develop skills for countering gender-based bullying or discrimination, strengthen "gender resilience," and manage non-gender-related sources of stress. Each individual's gender journey is unique, and therefore clinicians are advised to follow the child's or adolescent's lead without imposing one's own expectations for how the patient should ultimately identify in terms of gender. Prepubertal children may first be referred to psychotherapy to explore their gender identity. Therapists may help patients explore the range of possibilities for gender identity and expression and consider the relationship between gender identity and sexual orientation. A transgender or gender-diverse person may take steps toward becoming socially affirmed, such as going by a self-identified name and pronouns, as well as changing their gender expression and accessing other forms of nonmedical gender affirmation to more accurately reflect their gender identity. This affirmation process may take place gradually and should follow a child's or adolescent's wishes and level of comfort; for example, a transgender girl may initially feel more comfortable wearing a dress and make-up in the safety and comfort of her home rather than at school.

Legal gender affirmation is the recognition of a person's gender identity through legal recourse, and it may take place through a name or gender marker change on official government-issued documents, for example.

Gender minority stress can be distressing for both the child and their parent(s)/caregiver(s), who should receive education and guidance on how to best support their child in their gender journey. Of note, transgender and gender-diverse youth with unsupportive parents experience significantly greater depressive symptoms and past-year suicide attempts. In contrast, those endorsing high levels of family support have increased satisfaction with life, excellent mental health, high self-esteem, and adequate housing. Helpful resources for parents may include the following: the American Academy of Child and Adolescent Psychiatry (AACAP) Facts for Families article on transgender and gender diverse youth (https://www.aacap.org/AACAP/Families_and_Youth/Facts_for_Families/FFF-Guide/transgender-and-gender-diverse-youth-122.aspx) and the Human Rights Campaign resource packet for caregivers (https://www.hrc.org/resources/supporting-caring-for-transgender-children).

KEY POINTS TO REMEMBER

- Gender minority stress may arise when gender identity does not align with societal expectations based on the sex assigned at birth and is not fully affirmed.
- The primary approach to care for transgender and gender-diverse youth is gender affirmation, which may include psychological, social, legal, medical, or surgical affirmation.
- Gonadotropin-releasing hormone analogs for pubertal suppression can help by preventing harmful endogenous puberty and allowing more time for exploration of gender identity.
- Withholding gender-affirming medical care is not a neutral act and may cause significant harm.
- Empower children to explore their gender identity and follow their lead.

Further Reading

Human Rights Campaign. Supporting and Caring for Transgender Children. Retrieved May 27, 2020, from http://Hrc.org/resources/supporting-caring-for-transgenderchildren.

Perlson JE, Walters OC, Keuroghlian AS. Envisioning a future for transgender and gender-diverse people beyond the DSM. *Br J Psychiatry* 2020;25:1–2.

Ristori J, Steensma TD. Gender dysphoria in childhood. *Int Rev Psychiatry* 2016;28(1):13–20.

Spack NP, Edwards-Leeper L, Feldman HA, et al. Children and adolescents with gender identity disorder referred to a pediatric medical center. *Pediatrics* 2012;129(3):418–425.

Steensma TD, McGuire JK, Kreukels BP, et al. Factors associated with desistence and persistence of childhood gender dysphoria: A quantitative follow-up study. *J Am Acad Child Adolesc Psychiatry* 2013;52(6):582–590.

Travers R, Bauer, G, Pyne J. Impacts of strong parental support for trans youth: A report prepared for Children's Aid Society of Toronto and Delisle Youth Services. *Trans Pulse* 2012:1–5.

Turban JL, Carswell J, Keuroghlian AS. Understanding pediatric patients who discontinue gender-affirming hormonal interventions. *JAMA Pediatr* 2018;172(10):903–904.

Turban JL, Ehrensaft D. Gender identity in youth: Treatment paradigms and controversies. *J Child Psychol Psychiatry* 2018;59:1228–1243.

Vance SR, Ehrensaft D, Rosenthal SM. Psychology and medical care of gender nonconforming youth. *Pediatrics* 2014;134(6):1184–1192.

World Professional Association for Transgender Health. Standards of Care Version 7. Retrieved May 27, 2020, from http://Wpath.org/publications/soc.

27 An adolescent with binge drinking

Eun Kyung Ellen Kim and David L. Beckmann

A 17-year-old girl is referred to your psychiatry clinic by her pediatrician. During her annual wellness visit with her pediatrician, she reported consuming alcohol every weekend. Recently she has been drinking to the point of blacking out. Her grades have gone from straight Bs to Cs and she has been kicked off her school soccer team. She has been hiding her deteriorating school performance and alcohol use from her parents. Her pediatrician had advised her to quit drinking, but now, three months later, her pattern of alcohol use has not changed, and her grades have worsened, which prompted a psychiatry referral. In your interview, she says her drinking is not a problem but is open to drinking less frequently and asks for your guidance.

What Do You Do Now?

The pattern of disruption of normal functioning (declining school grades, quitting afterschool activities) and excessive alcohol consumption resulting in blackouts is highly concerning for alcohol use disorder (AUD). Alcohol use disorder is a chronic disorder, with a variable course typically including periods of remission and relapse, leading to clinically significant impairment or distress. It is important to screen for alcohol use in all adolescents, as it can lead to unintentional injuries, accidents, and death, as well as long-term disruptions in brain development. Persistent AUD can lead to significant cognitive, behavioral, and physiologic problems as well as social, economic, and sometimes legal consequences.

EPIDEMIOLOGY

The prevalence of AUD among adolescents (12 to 17 years old) is 4.6%, compared to 8.5% in adults (18 years and older). The age of onset of AUD peaks in the late teens to mid-20s, although alcohol-related problems that do not meet full criteria for AUD may occur in younger adolescents. Rates are highest among Hispanic (6%) and Native American and Alaska Natives (5.7%), followed by White (5%) adolescents. Risk factors for AUD include a family history of AUD (three to four times increased risk), environmental factors such as cultural attitudes and availability of alcohol, and early initiation of drinking. Common psychiatric comorbidities among adolescents with AUD include conduct disorder and other substance use disorders, as well as anxiety disorders and major depressive disorder.

SIGNS AND SYMPTOMS

The *Diagnostic and Statistical Manual of Mental Disorders*, Fifth Edition (DSM-5), describes 11 possible signs and symptoms of problematic alcohol use. The diagnosis of AUD requires that at least two of 11 factors are met; these factors can be categorized as factors relating to impaired control, social impairment, risky use, and physiological effects. The impaired control criteria (one through four) include using alcohol in larger amounts or over a longer period of time than was intended; a persistent desire or unsuccessful efforts to cut down or control alcohol use; a great deal of time spent obtaining, using, or recovering from alcohol;

and experiencing cravings, or a strong desire or urge to use alcohol. The social impairment criteria (five through seven) include recurrent alcohol use resulting in a failure to fulfill major role obligations at work, school, or home; continued alcohol use despite persistent or recurrent social or interpersonal problems; and reduction in important social, occupational, or recreational activities as a result of alcohol use. The risky use criteria (eight and nine) include recurrent alcohol use in physically hazardous situations and continued use despite knowledge of or having a persistent or recurrent physical or psychological problem that is likely to have been caused or exacerbated by alcohol. The physiological effects criteria (10 and 11) refer to alcohol tolerance or withdrawal. Tolerance is defined by either a need for markedly increased amounts of alcohol to achieve intoxication or a markedly diminished effect with continued use of the same amount of alcohol. Withdrawal manifests as alcohol withdrawal syndrome or the use of alcohol or a related substance (e.g., benzodiazepines) to relieve or avoid withdrawal symptoms.

The severity of AUD exists on a spectrum and is specified by the number of symptoms that are present: mild (two or three symptoms), moderate (four or five symptoms), and severe (six or more symptoms). Remission of AUD is defined as meeting none of the criteria for AUD for at least three months, aside from criterion four, "craving, or a strong desire or urge to use alcohol." Early remission is defined as meeting remission criteria for between three and 12 months, while sustained remission is defined as being in remission for more than 12 months.

Adolescent AUD differs from adult AUD in several ways. Alcohol consumption in adolescents is typically marked by episodic and binge drinking rather than drinking daily or most days. Healthy adolescent patients are also less likely to experience tolerance or withdrawal than adult patients. Interpersonal problems or failure to meet obligations may present differently in adolescents, for example, changing peer groups or declining grades. Adolescents are also more likely to engage in risk-taking behaviors related to substance use. Finally, a teenager's drinking may be problematic (e.g., drinking only occasionally but in unsafe situations) while not formally meeting criteria for the diagnosis of AUD. These patterns of problematic alcohol consumption also warrant screening, monitoring, and potential intervention.

ASSESSMENT

Before approaching the subject of alcohol use, the issue of confidentiality must be discussed between the adolescent patient and provider. Establishing confidentiality makes it more likely that adolescents will answer honestly, access care, and build a therapeutic alliance with the provider. However, breaching confidentiality is warranted if the adolescent is using alcohol in a way that poses acute safety concerns.

One useful approach to the delivery of early intervention and treatment to people with substance use disorders and those at risk of developing substance use disorders in the primary care setting is the Screening, Brief Intervention, and/or Referral to Treatment (SBIRT) model. In this model, screening assesses the severity of substance use and identifies the appropriate level of treatment; brief intervention focuses on increasing motivation toward behavioral change; and referral to treatment provides access to specialty care if needed. The National Institute on Alcohol Abuse and Alcoholism (NIAAA) Youth Guide suggests a two-question screening process, including asking about the adolescent's friends' drinking frequency and the patient's drinking frequency to stratify the patient's risk for AUD by age and frequency of alcohol use. If further assessment is warranted, the "Car, Relax, Alone, Forget, Friends, Trouble" (CRAFFT) screening tool is a well-validated assessment tool that can be used as an interview guide. A thorough substance use history should also inquire about the adolescent's drinking pattern, episodes of binge drinking, risky behavior (e.g., high-risk sexual activity, driving while intoxicated, etc.), and other substance use (particularly other sedatives like opiates and benzodiazepines). These questions should be asked in a nonjudgmental manner.

In terms of laboratory testing, the most direct test is blood alcohol concentration either via breathalyzer or a blood serum test. A urine or serum toxicology screen should be part of the formal evaluation and ongoing assessment to evaluate for co-occurring substance use, especially since combining alcohol with other substances, particularly sedatives, increases the risk of overdose. Gamma-glutamyl transferase (GGT) and carbohydrate-deficient transferrin (CDT) are sensitive markers for heavy alcohol consumption but are rarely useful in patients with a binge pattern of drinking, as is more common among adolescents. Liver function tests can reveal evidence of liver injury secondary to heavy drinking and should be checked prior to initiating certain pharmacological interventions (discussed later).

LEVEL OF CARE

There are many levels of care for AUD, ranging from outpatient care to inpatient residential treatment programs. Among outpatient programs, family therapy is the most well-validated approach. Individual therapy can involve different modalities such as motivational interviewing or cognitive behavioral therapy. Group therapy and peer support groups (teen Alcoholics Anonymous, Self-Management and Recovery Training [SMART] Recovery) are cost-effective approaches that encourage peer support.

Beyond these outpatient approaches, a partial hospitalization program can offer short-term, more intensive outpatient treatment for patients with co-occurring substance use and mental health disorders. Residential treatment provides structured, live-in environments to patients with severe substance use disorders with or without co-occurring psychiatric disorders. Inpatient programs are short term and typically only used when there is concern for withdrawal or acute risk of harm (e.g., suicidality).

BIOLOGICAL TREATMENT

Evidence for the use of medication-assisted treatment for AUD, while commonly used in the adult population, is limited in adolescents. Naltrexone is an opioid antagonist that works to reduce the craving for alcohol. It is the most commonly prescribed medication to treat AUD in adolescents due to its tolerability and relative safety. This medication can be started while the patient is still drinking but is contraindicated if the patient has hepatitis or liver failure. Liver function tests should be checked prior to starting the medication and periodically after starting the medication. Acamprosate, a glutamate receptor modulator, is also used to reduce cravings and is appropriate in patients with pre-existing liver problems but is contraindicated in those with severe kidney impairment. Its three-times-daily dosing may make adherence more difficult. Finally, disulfiram is primarily used to prevent alcohol consumption. The medication works by altering alcohol metabolism to cause a buildup of acetaldehyde, a mild toxin that produces an acute sensitivity to alcohol characterized by flushing, a throbbing headache, vertigo, hypotension, nausea, vomiting, and sweating. Importantly, this medication only works if the patient is adherent to it and is best used in highly motivated patients after an extended period of abstinence.

PSYCHOSOCIAL TREATMENT

Treatment of AUD warrants a multimodal approach that can be tailored based on the severity of the disorder. Typically, during time-limited encounters such as an outpatient pediatrics visit, a patient with mild to moderate AUD is given clear and brief advice to quit, encouraged to set a goal to quit or reduce alcohol use, and referred to substance use–targeted counseling if unable to meet the identified goal. Patients with severe AUD are referred to psychiatrists for a comprehensive biopsychosocial assessment and to assess for the presence of comorbid psychiatric disorders.

Once in the psychiatric setting, the first step is to use a motivational interviewing (MI) approach to start a conversation about changing alcohol use. Motivational interviewing is a collaborative counseling approach that aims to resolve ambivalence and strengthen motivation to elicit a patient-driven behavioral change. As the most evidence-based approach, MI gains patient buy-in and builds rapport while progressively working toward harm reduction or abstinence. While MI does not condone problematic drinking, it eschews a directive approach—which adolescents often reject—in favor of working with the patient's own goals and motivations.

Finally, family or parental involvement is an essential part of AUD treatment, regardless of the adolescent's degree of participation. Family interventions provide opportunities for psychoeducation and encourage the adolescent to seek appropriate treatment and abstinence. Parental involvement also allows for effective contingency planning; for example, parents can be counseled to limit access to the family car if the patient does not engage in treatment. Caregivers can be referred to the American Academy of Child and Adolescent Psychiatry (AACAP) Facts for Families guide on alcohol use in teens (https://www.aacap.org/AACAP/Families_and_Youth/Facts_for_Families/FFF-Guide/Teens-Alcohol-And-Other-Drugs-003.aspx).

- Alcohol use disorder affects about 5% of adolescents.
- All adolescents should be screened for alcohol and other substance use after discussing confidentiality.
- Use a motivational interviewing approach to discuss alcohol use and encourage harm reduction or abstinence.
- Treatment should include individual and family therapy; medications may be a useful adjunct.
- Parental/family involvement in the treatment of AUD in adolescents is essential.

Further Reading

Bukstein OG, Bernet W, Arnold V, et al. Practice parameter for the assessment and treatment of children and adolescents with substance use disorders. *J Am Acad Child Adolesc Psychiatry* 2005;44(6):609–621.

Center for Substance Abuse Treatment. (1999). *Enhancing Motivation for Change in Substance Abuse Treatment.* Substance Abuse and Mental Health Services Administration (US). http://www.ncbi.nlm.nih.gov/books/NBK64967/.

Levy SJL, Williams JF, Committee on Substance Use and Prevention. Substance use screening, brief intervention, and referral to treatment. *Pediatrics* 2016;138(1):e20161211.

National Institute on Alcohol Abuse and Alcoholism (NIAAA). *Alcohol Screening and Brief Intervention for Youth: A Practitioner's Guide.* January 6, 2012. https://www.niaaa.nih.gov/publications/clinical-guides-and-manuals/ alcohol-screening-and-brief-intervention-youth.

Ryan SA, Kokotailo P, Committee on Substance Use and Prevention. Alcohol use by youth. *Pediatrics* 2019;144(1):e20191357.

28 An adolescent with new-onset inattention

Samantha M. Taylor and
David L. Beckmann

A 16-year-old male is brought to a psychiatry clinic by
his mother due to new concerns related to focus and
concentration. His grades have fallen in the last year and he
quit the swim team. His mother is worried that he is showing
signs of attention-deficit/hyperactivity disorder (ADHD) and
asks if he should be started on a stimulant medication. She
notes that he has also been more irritable and withdrawn
lately.

On initial evaluation, the patient reports his mood is
"pretty good" but notes difficulty with concentrating in school
over the last year. He denies auditory or visual hallucinations
as well as suicidal or homicidal ideation. When you ask about
substance use, he endorses smoking increasing amounts
of cannabis daily over the past 18 months with his friends,
including before and during school. He denies any other
substance use. He is amenable to urine drug testing today in
clinic but asks you not to disclose the results to his mother.

What Do You Do Now?

The patient's noted behavioral changes and functional decline in school over the last year in the setting of daily cannabis use are concerning for cannabis use disorder. Given his prior academic success without a history of learning difficulties, it is unlikely that the patient has ADHD, which, according to the *Diagnostic and Statistical Manual of Mental Disorders*, Fifth Edition (DSM-5) criteria, requires symptoms to begin prior to the age of 12 years and not be better explained by another mental disorder including substance intoxication or withdrawal.

Evidence demonstrates that acute cannabis use is associated with impaired cognitive function in a dose-dependent manner, particularly in the domains of attention, concentration, memory, and learning. Long-term cognitive effects include impaired verbal memory and cognitive processing speed, though these can be reversed with abstinence from cannabis use. Even one week of abstinence may result in significant improvements in cognitive functioning. Cannabis can transiently cause symptoms of psychosis in some users. There is increasing evidence that chronic cannabis use, particularly daily use of products with high concentrations of tetrahydrocannabinol (THC), is causatively associated with the development of schizophrenia. Other commonly occurring co-morbid psychiatric disorders include major depressive disorder, bipolar disorder, anxiety disorders, and personality disorders. Individuals who use cannabis are at increased risk of accidental death by injury or motor vehicle collisions. Medical complications of cannabis use include peri-odontal disease (due to decreased saliva production and an association with poorer dental care), cannabis hyperemesis syndrome, and decreased sperm count.

EPIDEMIOLOGY

Cannabis is the second most commonly used psychoactive substance in the world across all age groups after alcohol. The primary psychoactive substance in cannabis is THC. In the United States, three million people aged 12 years or older initiated cannabis use in 2017. In 2019, 11.8% of eighth graders, 28.8% of 10th graders, and 35.7% of 12th graders reported cannabis use over the last year. While yearly use of cannabis from 2018 to 2019 among teens has remained stable overall, national trends suggest daily marijuana use amongst eighth and 10th graders has increased dramatically, by 85.7% and 41.2%, respectively, compared to 2018.

SIGNS AND SYMPTOMS

Patients who are acutely intoxicated with cannabis will often describe feeling "high" or euphoric, although observers may note decreased alertness. Some patients experience reductions in anxiety, while others report increased anxiety, dysphoria, and panic symptoms. Risk factors for these negative experiences include first-time cannabis use, underlying anxiety disorders, and overingestion of edible cannabis products. High doses of THC-potent cannabis can cause psychotic or manic symptoms including bizarre behavior, grandiosity, paranoia, magical thinking, and auditory or visual hallucinations. Cognitively, acute cannabis intoxication slows reaction time and impairs attention, concentration, short-term memory, and judgment. Psychomotor impairment lasts for up to 12 to 24 hours after last cannabis use due to the accumulation of THC in adipose tissues. Other symptoms of acute cannabis intoxication may include tachycardia, hypertension, hyperventilation, conjunctival injection, dry mouth, increased appetite, nystagmus, ataxia, and slurred speech. In young children naive to cannabis and more prone to accidental overdose, neurologic symptoms such as ataxia, hyperkinesis, and marked lethargy may be more prominent.

Cannabis use disorder is defined by the DSM-5 as a problematic pattern of cannabis use that leads to clinically significant impairment or marked distress manifested by at least two of the following symptoms within a 12-month period of time: (1) cannabis is often taken in larger amounts or over a longer period of time than intended; (2) persistent desire or unsuccessful efforts to cut down or control cannabis use; (3) a great deal of time is spent engaging in activities necessary to obtain cannabis, use cannabis, or recover from its effects; (4) craving, or a strong desire or urge to use; (5) recurrent cannabis use resulting in a failure to fulfill major role obligations at work, school, or home; (6) continued cannabis use despite having persistent or recurrent social or interpersonal problems caused or exacerbated by the effects of cannabis; (7) important social, occupational, or recreational activities are given up or reduced because of cannabis use; (8) recurrent use in situations in which it is physically hazardous (e.g., driving); (9) cannabis use is continued despite knowledge of having a persistent or recurrent physical or psychological problem that is likely to have been caused or exacerbated by cannabis use; (10) tolerance defined by a need for increased amounts of cannabis to achieve intoxication/desired effect and/or markedly diminished effect with continued use of the same amount of cannabis; and (11) withdrawal, as manifested by the characteristic withdrawal syndrome and/or cannabis use to relieve or avoid withdrawal symptoms.

Specifiers are included to indicate remission status and severity. The remission status options include "in early remission," defined as meeting none of the cannabis use disorder criteria aside from craving, for at least three months but for less than 12 months, and "in sustained remission," where remission has been achieved for 12 months or longer. The specifier "in a controlled environment" is used if the individual is in an environment where access to cannabis is restricted. Finally, the severity specifiers are used to indicate the number of symptoms that are present: "mild" (two to three symptoms), "moderate" (four to five symptoms), and "severe" (six or more symptoms).

The DSM-5 criteria for cannabis withdrawal requires cannabis use to have been heavy and prolonged, defined as daily or nearly daily use, over a period of months with three or more of the following symptoms within one week of cessation of use: (1) irritability, anger, or aggression; (2) nervousness or anxiety; (3) sleep difficulty; (4) decreased appetite or weight loss; (5) restlessness; (6) depressed mood; and (7) abdominal pain, shakiness/tremors, sweating, fever, chills, or headache.

ASSESSMENT

Screening for substance use in adolescents, specifically cannabis use, can be conducted by any clinician. A nonjudgmental approach to discussing substance use with patients is always recommended. Self-reported screening is the most commonly used method for ascertaining cannabis use among adolescents. Simply asking the patient in private how many times in the past year the individual has used cannabis has been shown to have fairly high sensitivity and specificity. If the patient endorses cannabis use, a brief intervention should be conducted consisting of a discussion of patterns of substance use, risks of using the substance, and motivation for discontinuation.

If confirming cannabis use is imperative, patient self-report is less sensitive than toxicology screening, which is typically conducted with urine screens, although saliva, blood, and hair assays also exist. Urine screens are more subject to false positives than false negatives and thus may need to be confirmed by a more specific test if there is discrepancy between reported use and the toxicology results. Of note, THC is rapidly absorbed and stored in adipose tissue, leading to a slow release of THC into the bloodstream over time. As such, drug testing for THC in urine does not necessarily correlate with recency of use and THC concentrations in the blood and urine are often not linked to clinical symptomatology. Clinically, however, quantitative THC levels can be useful to clarify extremes of use (i.e., if the level is very high or very low) and are a reasonable, though imperfect, proxy for monitoring for changes in use (once corrected for urine concentration by obtaining a urine creatinine).

With regard to the aforementioned case, a urine toxicology screen may be obtained to confirm this patient's reported cannabis use and rule out other simultaneous substance use. The patient should be encouraged to discuss his substance use with his mother, though required disclosure to parents by physicians varies by state. The psychiatrist may offer to be a liaison between the patient and his mother to discuss his substance use.

Ideally, patient assent should be obtained before drug testing, as mandatory reporting to guardians of adolescent substance use also varies by state. Confidentiality should be honored whenever possible, and limits to confidentiality should be clearly explained in advance of drug testing to the patient. Research demonstrates that when adolescents perceive that health care services are not confidential, they are less likely to seek care. Notably, if a patient presents with acutely altered mental status in the emergency room and is felt to be at imminent medical risk, drug testing to rule out substance use would be considered ethically appropriate.

LEVEL OF CARE

Most cases of cannabis use disorder can be managed in the outpatient setting and do not require inpatient psychiatric admission. Exceptions to this may include instances where intoxicated patients, despite adequate observation time in the emergency department, continue to demonstrate symptoms of psychosis.

In cases of persistent or severe psychosis in patients who endorse only using cannabis, the presence of a primary psychotic disorder should be considered. Clinicians should also have a high index of suspicion for synthetic cannabinoid use that is not detected on routine urine drug testing. Synthetic cannabinoids bind to cannabinoid receptors with significantly higher affinity than THC in natural cannabis, leading to the possibility of severe intoxication and withdrawal syndromes including sustained psychotic symptoms and seizures, respectively.

BIOLOGICAL TREATMENT

There are currently no Food and Drug Administration (FDA)-approved medications for cannabis use disorder in adolescents or adults. Two randomized controlled trials have demonstrated that N-acetylcysteine (NAC), an antioxidant precursor to glutathione, is superior to placebo for diminishing cravings and reducing the risk of relapse in adolescents with cannabis use disorder. A suggested safe and potentially efficacious dosage of NAC for the treatment of cannabis use disorder is 1,200 mg twice daily for four to eight weeks. In patients with severe anxiety, psychosis, or agitation, atypical antipsychotics and/or benzodiazepines may be considered at the lowest effective doses for symptomatic treatment. Use of these agents is typically reserved for the emergency room or inpatient psychiatric unit settings and should be discontinued prior to discharge. Management of cannabis use–related side effects such as difficulty with concentration or focus should be addressed by reducing and/or eliminating cannabis use. If symptoms of inattention persist after discontinuation of cannabis use, stimulant medications should be used only after carefully considering the increased risk of stimulant medication misuse.

PSYCHOSOCIAL TREATMENT

The most effective evidence-based therapy modalities for cannabis use disorder treatment include motivational enhancement therapy, contingency management, cognitive behavioral therapy, and a variety of family-based therapies. Which therapy modality is selected is often based on availability, patient preference, and the likelihood of adherence. Motivational enhancement therapy focuses on helping patients resolve their ambivalence about engaging in treatment and stopping their drug use. Contingency management focuses on providing the patient tangible rewards as reinforcement for target behaviors such as abstinence or reduced substance use. Cognitive behavioral therapy focuses on improving the patient's understanding of the dynamic interplay between their thoughts, feelings, and behaviors with the goal of learning effective coping skills to replace substance use.

Family-based therapies focus on engaging parents and siblings in addressing the adolescent's substance use with an added focus on how family dynamics may contribute to substance use. Notably, involvement of family in some capacity is considered pivotal to improved outcomes, as adolescents are subject to parental rules, controls, and supports. Parent coaching therefore plays a crucial role in promoting successful adherence to the patient's substance use–related goals. Parents can be referred to the American Academy of Child and Adolescent Psychiatry Facts for Families article on teenage marijuana use (https://www.aacap.org/AACAP/Families_and_Youth/Facts_for_Families/FFF-Guide/Marijuana-and-Teens-106.aspx).

Finally, while the long-term goal of substance use treatment in adolescents is often abstinence, it may be most effective to begin with harm reduction strategies. These may include trying to reduce use and/or avoid adverse consequences of use such as driving while intoxicated or using cannabis during school hours. Beginning with a harm reduction approach may promote an improved patient-physician relationship through allowing the patient to build motivation to change substance use patterns over time, while targeting the most severe psychosocial impairments of the substance use.

KEY POINTS TO REMEMBER

- Cannabis is second only to alcohol as the most commonly used psychoactive substance by adolescents.
- Cannabis use disorder is associated with significant impairments in multiple cognitive domains; however,

improvements may be seen in as little as one week with sustained abstinence.
- Heavy use of large amounts of THC during adolescence increases the likelihood of developing schizophrenia.
- Synthetic cannabinoids are chemically different from those found in the marijuana plant and can lead to severe psychotic episodes. They are not detected with routine THC drug screening.
- Tetrahydrocannabinol is stored in adipose tissues and therefore often remains in enterohepatic circulation beyond periods of acute intoxication or withdrawal.
- There are currently no FDA-approved medications for cannabis use disorder; however, NAC has demonstrated efficacy in reducing cravings and risk of relapse in randomized controlled trials.

Further Reading

National Institute on Drug Abuse. *Principles of Drug Addiction Treatment: A Research-Based Guide.* 3rd ed. January 17, 2018. Retrieved April 20, 2020, from https://www.drugabuse.gov/publications/principles-drug-addiction-treatment-research-based-guide-third-edition.

National Institute on Drug Abuse, National Institutes of Health, U.S. Department of Health and Human Services. Monitoring the Future Survey: High School and Youth Trends 2019. December 2019.

Tomko RL, Jones JL, Gilmore AK, et al. N-acetylcysteine: A potential treatment for substance use disorders. *Curr Psychiatry* 2018;17(6):30–55.

Weddle M, Kokotailo PK. Confidentiality and consent in adolescent substance abuse: An update. *Virtual Mentor* 2005;7(3):239–243.

29 Confusion and mental status changes in a medically ill child

Robyn P. Thom

A 13-year-old girl is admitted to the intensive care unit for management of third-degree burns including airway burns due to a house fire. She was intubated for airway protection and her course was complicated by septic shock and acute kidney injury. Upon extubation, the pediatric psychiatry consultation-liaison team is consulted due to concerns regarding tearfulness, impaired sleep, and reduced participation in physical therapy.

On assessment, she is tearful, disoriented, and inattentive. She frequently asks for you to repeat your questions, takes a long time to respond to questions, and cannot articulate why she is crying. She cannot register the three words that you ask her to remember. Nursing staff note that she has been asleep for most of the day but is restless at night, rarely asleep. She has no history of significant medical conditions or emotional concerns. While in the hospital, she has had some periods of increased lucidity, during which she expresses fear and confusion about her circumstances.

What Do You Do Now?

The patient is suffering from delirium, an acute transient syndrome of global brain dysfunction, that is the pathophysiological consequence of an underlying medical condition or toxic exposure. Early identification and management of delirium are important because it contributes to increased mortality, is associated with poor long-term functional outcomes, results in higher health care costs, disrupts provision of medical care, and can cause high levels of patient and family distress.

EPIDEMIOLOGY

Delirium is becoming increasingly recognized in the pediatric population. Reported prevalence rates range from 13% to 44% of hospitalized children, depending on the age and illness severity. The prevalence of delirium in pediatric critical care settings is 20% to 30%. Risk factors for pediatric delirium include younger age (0 to 5 years), developmental delay (3.5 times increased risk), multiorgan illness, use of deliriogenic medication classes (opioids, benzodiazepines, anticholinergic medications), and mechanical ventilation.

SIGNS AND SYMPTOMS

According to the *Diagnostic and Statistical Manual of Mental Disorders*, Fifth Edition (DSM-5), delirium is characterized by a disturbance in attention, awareness, and cognition that develops over a short period of time (hours to days) and fluctuates in severity. Domains of cognition that can be affected include memory, orientation, language, visuospatial ability, and perception. The disturbance is the direct pathophysiological consequence of another medical condition, substance intoxication, or withdrawal. Patients with a severely reduced level of arousal such as coma are excluded from the diagnosis.

Additional features of delirium include altered sleep cycle, changes in affect, and psychomotor disturbance. Motoric subtypes of delirium include hyperactive, hypoactive, and mixed level of activity. Hyperactive delirium is characterized by psychomotor agitation, restlessness, and emotional lability. Hypoactive delirium is characterized by psychomotor retardation, lethargy, and decreased arousal. Mixed delirium presents with either a normal level of psychomotor activity or fluctuations in activity level. Clinical features of delirium that are more common in children than adults include irritability, affective lability, agitation, sleep-wake disturbance, and fluctuating symptoms. Unique characteristics of pediatric delirium include developmental regression, inconsolability by the caregiver, and reduced eye contact with the caregiver. Delusions and hallucinations are less common in pediatric delirium than in adult delirium.

ASSESSMENT

There are no laboratory tests or biomarkers with high sensitivity or specificity for delirium, and a thorough clinical evaluation is the gold standard for diagnosis. Repeated evaluations and collaboration with multidisciplinary team members including nursing, the primary medical team, and child-life specialists can be helpful to determine whether symptoms fluctuate over time. Obtaining information from the child's parent/caregiver about the child's baseline cognitive and attentional functioning, unusual behaviors, emotional changes, perceptual disturbances, and altered interpersonal interactions will help inform the diagnosis. Assessing for the presence of DSM-5 criteria for delirium in children requires a developmental approach, since a child's ability to sustain attention and engage in cognitively complex tasks progresses to adult levels over time. Features of the mental status examination that occur in delirium include evidence of confusion and abnormal engagement, change in psychomotor activity, decreased eye contact, affective lability or incongruence, incoherent thought process or slowed processing, and perceptual disturbances. Cognitive changes include lack of orientation, memory disturbance, and decreased level of consciousness. Bedside cognition can be assessed in older children using the Montreal Cognitive Assessment (MoCA). There are several delirium rating scales that have been validated in the pediatric population. The most widely used scales are the Pediatric Confusion Assessment Method for the Intensive Care Unit (PCAM-ICU) and the Columbia Assessment for Pediatric Delirium (CAPD).

Patients with suspected delirium should undergo a physical examination and laboratory investigation to determine potential underlying medical etiologies. Screening laboratory tests should include a complete blood count, metabolic panel, and urinalysis. If there are localizing neurologic signs, neuroimaging should be obtained. Further workup would depend on the patient's clinical presentation and the results of screening laboratory tests.

The differential diagnosis for delirium can be broad since symptoms of delirium can be highly variable and mimic other psychiatric disorders including depression, mania, and primary psychotic disorders. Distinguishing features of delirium that are usually not present in primary mood or psychotic disorders include the abrupt onset of symptoms, fluctuation of symptoms, impaired orientation and awareness, and evidence of medical illness. It is also important to distinguish delirium from catatonia, as this would affect the treatment approach.

PREVENTION

Multimodal nonpharmacologic delirium prevention protocols have been demonstrated to decrease the incidence of delirium in various adult settings including general medicine units, intensive care units, and nursing homes. Common features of delirium prevention programs include improving orientation, early mobilization, sleep-wake cycle preservation, addressing sensory needs, minimizing use of physical restraints, and optimizing nutrition and hydration status. Although these protocols have not been studied in pediatric populations, adaptation of these strategies may also be helpful in preventing and treating delirium in children.

BIOLOGICAL TREATMENT

The primary treatment of delirium is identification and management of the underlying medical etiologies. The most common medical etiologies of delirium in children include infection, medication-related factors, and autoimmune conditions. Common classes of deliriogenic medications include anticholinergic medications, benzodiazepines, and opioids. These medications should be minimized, substituted, or tapered as medically appropriate. Supportive treatments include adequate pain management, nutrition optimization, early mobilization, and prevention of deep venous thrombosis.

There are no Food and Drug Administration (FDA)-approved medications for the treatment of delirium in either adults or children. Antipsychotics are the most widely used class of medications to manage symptoms that threaten safety or impede the provision of medical care. Antipsychotic treatment targets include agitation, paranoia, and hallucinations; however, there is no evidence that antipsychotics impact the core attentional or cognitive symptoms of delirium. Both first- and second-generation antipsychotics have been used in this setting. The lowest effective dose should be used to minimize the risk of side effects, and antipsychotics should be tapered prior to discharge.

PSYCHOSOCIAL TREATMENT

Delirium can be distressing for both the child and their parents. Parents should receive psychoeducation regarding the presenting symptoms, typical course, and management of delirium. The American Academy of Child and Adolescent Psychiatry (AACAP) has published a Facts for Families article on delirium (https://www.aacap.org/App_Themes/AACAP/docs/homepage/headlines/2015/DeliriumFlyer.AACAP.pdf), which can be distributed to parents. Parents can help their child with delirium by being present at the bedside, offering distraction with familiar or comforting objects such as a favorite toy or music, helping the team identify symptoms of delirium, and promoting daytime activity and nighttime sleep.

Hospitalized children with delirium may benefit from supportive psychotherapy at the bedside and involvement with child-life specialists as well as other stress reduction strategies such as pet therapy, music therapy, or art therapy. After delirium has resolved, it may be helpful to use simple language to explain delirium. Patients should also receive screening and assessment for the development of secondary mood, anxiety, or posttraumatic stress disorder symptoms upon discharge.

KEY POINTS TO REMEMBER

- Pediatric delirium occurs in 20% to 30% of hospitalized critically ill children.
- Hallmarks of pediatric delirium include irritability, affective lability, agitation, sleep-wake cycle disturbance, and fluctuation of symptoms.

- Pediatric delirium should be considered in the "inconsolable" or "nonsedatable" child.
- The primary treatment of delirium is identification and management of the underlying medical etiologies.
- Time-limited use of antipsychotics may be considered for management of symptoms that pose a safety concern, impede provision of medical care, or cause high levels of patient distress.

Further Reading

Bourgeois JA, ed. *Delirium: Prevention, Symptoms, and Treatment.* New York: Nova Science Publishers, 2017.

Schieveld JNM, Janssen NJJF. Delirium in the pediatric patient: On the growing awareness of its clinical interdisciplinary importance. *JAMA Pediatr* 2014;168(7):595–596.

Thom RP, Levy-Carrick NC, Bui MP, et al. Delirium. *Am J Psychiatry* 2019;176(10):785–792.

Traube C, Silver G, Kearney J, et al. Cornell assessment of pediatric delirium: A valid, rapid, observational tool for screening delirium in the PICU. *Pediatr Crit Care Med* 2014;42(3):656–663.

Turkel SB, Jacobson J, Munzig E, et al. Atypical antipsychotic medications to control symptoms of delirium in children and adolescents. *J Child Adolesc Psychopharmacol* 2012;22(2):126–130.

Index

For the benefit of digital users, indexed terms that span two pages (e.g., 52–53) may, on occasion, appear on only one of those pages.

comprehensive behavioral intervention for tics (CBIT), 41
compulsions, 138–39. *See also* obsessive-compulsive disorder
confidentiality, 216, 225
constipation, 197–202
contingency management, 226–27
counseling, gender-affirming, 206
CPS (collaborative problem solving), 76

DBT. *See* dialectical behavior therapy
delirium, 229–34
depersonalization, 112–13
depression, 55–56
derealization, 112–13
developmental delays, 17–23
dialectical behavior therapy (DBT)
　for bipolar disorder, 68–69
　for disruptive mood dysregulation disorder (DMDD), 76–77
disinhibited social engagement disorder (DSED), 143–48
disruptive mood dysregulation disorder (DMDD), 71–78
disulfiram, 217–18
DSED (disinhibited social engagement disorder), 143–48
duloxetine, 124
dyscalculia, 13
dysgraphia, 13
dyslexia, 13

early-onset schizophrenia (EOS), 44–45, 46
eating disorders
　anorexia nervosa (AN), 181–87
　avoidant/restrictive food intake disorder (ARFID), 175–80
　bulimia nervosa (BN), 189–96
elimination disorders, 197–202
encopresis, 198–99
　functional, 198, 199–201
　organic, 199–200
ERP (exposure response prevention), 141

explosiveness. *See* disruptive mood dysregulation disorder (DMDD)
exposure response prevention (ERP), 141
exposure therapy
　for avoidant/restrictive food intake disorder (ARFID), 178–79
　for obsessive-compulsive disorder, 141
　for separation anxiety disorder (SAD), 100
　for social anxiety disorder (SAD), 107–8
　for specific phobias, 91–92
extrapyramidal symptoms (EPS), 49–50, 67–68

factitious disorder imposed on another (FDIA), 167–73
family-based therapy
　for anorexia nervosa (AN), 185–86
　for cannabis use disorder, 226–27
　for separation anxiety disorder (SAD), 100
family support groups, 141
FDIA (factitious disorder imposed on another), 167–73
fear. *See* phobia
fluoxetine
　for bulimia nervosa (BN), 193
　for obsessive-compulsive disorder (OCD), 140–41
　for selective mutism (SM), 83
fluvoxamine, 140–41
food avoidance. *See* avoidant/restrictive food intake disorder (ARFID)
Fragile X syndrome (FXS), 17–23
functional encopresis, 197–202

GAD (generalized anxiety disorder), 119–27
gender affirmation, 206–8
　discontinued experiences, 208–9
　legal, 210
gender-affirming counseling, 206
gender-affirming hormone therapy, 207–8
gender-affirming surgery, 206, 207–8